Smart Calories and Common Sense

Smart Calories and Common Sense

An Evidence-Based Guide to Indian Diets

Dr Anoop Misra

BLOOMSBURY
NEW DELHI • LONDON • OXFORD • NEW YORK • SYDNEY

BLOOMSBURY INDIA
Bloomsbury Publishing India Pvt. Ltd
Second Floor, LSC Building No. 4, DDA Complex, Pocket C – 6 & 7,
Vasant Kunj, New Delhi, 110070

BLOOMSBURY, BLOOMSBURY INDIA and the Diana logo
are trademarks of Bloomsbury Publishing Plc

First published in India 2026

ISBN: PB: 978-93-61317-15-6; eBook: 978-93-61311-68-0

2 4 6 8 10 9 7 5 3 1

For sale in the Indian subcontinent only
Typeset in Bembo by Manipal Technologies Limited
Printed and bound in India by Gopsons Papers Pvt. Ltd., Noida

FSC
www.fsc.org
MIX
Paper | Supporting responsible forestry
FSC® C191020

Disclaimer

The information provided in *Smart Calories and Common Sense* is intended for educational and informational purposes only. While every effort has been made to ensure the accuracy and timeliness of the content, readers should be aware of the following:

Evolution of Science: The nutritional studies and clinical data cited are updated as of the time of publication. However, nutritional science is a rapidly evolving field; new research may emerge that modifies or supersedes existing findings.

Nutritional Variability: Data regarding nutrient quality and content are derived from the most reliable scientific sources. These values should be viewed as estimates, as actual nutrient density may vary significantly based on analytical methods, geographical origin, storage and methods of preparation. Readers may encounter differing values across various databases and literature.

References: We have endeavoured to provide the best possible references for key facts and figures. Due to space constraints and the breadth of the subject matter, it is not feasible to provide an exhaustive list of every source consulted.

Evidence vs Myth: All statements are rooted in rigorous evidence-based science. Consequently, the information herein may contradict popular diet trends or 'health myths' circulating on social media. Many such viral claims lack scientific validation and may be incorrect or misleading.

Medical Advice: This book is not a substitute for professional medical advice, diagnosis or treatment. Always seek the advice of a physician or qualified nutritionist regarding a medical condition or before making significant changes to your diet or lifestyle.

Disclaimer

To my mother, Vidya Misra—ever remembered, ever cherished
To my wife, Angeli—my steadfast rock
To my children, Tanvi, Utkarsh and Daniel—endless love, endless joy

Nutrition relies on scientific facts, not on opinions, whims or unsubstantiated beliefs.

Contents

Tables

Easy Readings

Abbreviations

BMI	Body Mass Index
DASH	Dietary Approaches to Stop Hypertension
DHA	Docosahexaenoic Acid
EGCG	Epigallocatechin-3-Gallate
EN	Enteral Nutrition
FDA	Food and Drug Administration
GI	Glycaemic Index
GIP	Glucose-Dependent Insulinotropic Polypeptide
GL	Glycaemic Load
GLP-1 RA	Glucagon-Like Peptide-1 Receptor Agonists
GRAS	Generally Recognised As Safe
HDL	High-Density Lipoprotein
HFCS	High-Fructose Corn Syrup
HPMR	High-Protein Meal Replacement
IBS	Irritable Bowel Syndrome
ICMR	Indian Council of Medical Research
ICU	Intensive Care Unit
LDL	Low-Density Lipoprotein
MASLD	Metabolic Dysfunction-Associated Steatotic Liver Disease
MCT	Medium-Chain Triglycerides
MUFA	Monounsaturated Fatty Acid
NDOC	National Diabetes Obesity and Cholesterol Foundation
NNS	Non-Nutritive Sweetener
ONS	Oral Nutritional Supplements
PACER	High-Protein Complete Vegetarian Diets
PN	Parenteral Nutrition
PUFA	Polyunsaturated Fatty Acid
RDA	Recommended Dietary Allowances
SSB	Sugar-Sweetened Beverage
WHO	World Health Organization

Preface

In April 2020, confined at home during the COVID-19 lockdown, I suddenly found myself with an abundance of time. I began searching for a scientifically sound, India-centric book on diet. Surprisingly, I could not find one. That search gradually turned into resolve—to write a diet book grounded in science and relevant to Indian realities. Almost six years on, here we are.

Many diet books are available in India—so many that almost every food item has been hailed as a 'superfood' in one book and condemned as a 'silent killer' in another. Dietary myths circulate freely on social media, during morning walks and exercise groups, and at social gatherings, often passed down as grandmother's tales or repackaged as innovative but incorrect 'new science'. It is therefore not surprising that a ten-minute walk in the park can expose one to more dietary advice than a year of medical training. As a doctor, I often find myself spending more time correcting dietary misinformation than treating disease itself.

Most diet books, and much of this advice, are based on personal experiences, opinions, anecdotes or popular beliefs rather than rigorous science. While such narratives can be interesting and reassuring, they often lack consistency, reproducibility and—most importantly—evidence. This has led to considerable confusion among readers, patients and even health professionals about what truly constitutes a healthy diet.

Nutrition, at its core, is a science. Dietary advice must therefore rest on data, clinical studies and well-established physiological principles, not on trends, celebrity endorsements or isolated success stories. Unfortunately, evidence-based nutrition literature written specifically for the Indian context remains limited.

This book attempts to bridge that gap. It is firmly grounded in scientific evidence, drawing upon national and international guidelines, clinical research and decades of collective experience in metabolic health. At the same time, it deliberately avoids unnecessary technical complexity, making it accessible to laypersons who wish to make informed, sensible food choices. Equally, it serves as a reliable, fact-based reference for nutritionists, physicians, students and researchers. The aim is simple: to replace confusion with clarity, myths with data and opinions with evidence—so that dietary decisions are guided by common sense supported by science.

The book also critically examines many popular and often controversial dietary topics that dominate public discourse. These include intermittent fasting, ketogenic diets, diabetes reversal, weight-loss diets and the emerging role of weight-loss drugs, with a balanced discussion of their benefits, limitations, risks and suitability for Indians. Commonly debated foods such as mangoes and other fruits, nuts, dried fruits, honey, dates and spices like cinnamon are analysed using nutritional data rather than assumptions or popular beliefs. Staple foods such as wheat, rice and millets, different edible oils, fish and fish oils are evaluated for their effects on diabetes, obesity, heart disease, brain health, skin health, longevity and weight management.

To make complex science easier to digest, the book includes eighteen sections titled 'Easy Reading', which address practical and frequently asked questions—such as 'gluten-free diets', 'Do I need supplements?' and other everyday dilemmas—in a simple, relatable and clinically sound manner.

Importantly, many recommendations in this book are supported by published data, including several derived from our own research over the past two decades. This ensures that the guidance provided is scientifically robust, clinically relevant and culturally appropriate. Throughout, the emphasis remains on evidence, portion size, frequency, methods of preparation and overall dietary patterns, rather than on labelling foods as universally 'good' or 'bad'.

Ultimately, this book does not tell you what to believe—it helps you understand *why*. In doing so, it empowers readers to make informed, rational and sustainable dietary choices in an age crowded with noise, myths and misinformation.

In an age of viral 'new' diets, blatantly false WhatsApp messages and ever louder, often wrong opinions, this book recommends something refreshingly old-fashioned (but firmly rooted in solid evidence): Smart Calories and Common Sense.

1

What Is a Healthy Diet?

A healthy diet is one that provides the body with essential nutrition: fluids, macronutrients (carbohydrates, proteins, fats), micronutrients (vitamins, minerals) and adequate calories. It is balanced and diverse, comprising a variety of foods from different food groups in appropriate proportions. A healthy diet promotes overall well-being, supports optimal body function, aids in disease prevention, helps maintain a healthy weight and protects against diabetes, heart disease, hypertension, cholesterol disorders, fatty liver, cancers and multiple other disorders.[1 2 3]

Here is a more detailed breakdown:

Balance: A healthy diet includes a balance of carbohydrates, proteins and fats. Carbohydrates provide energy, proteins support tissue repair and growth, and fats are essential for hormone production and absorption of fat-soluble vitamins.

Variety: Consuming a variety of foods, such as fruits, vegetables, whole grains, lean proteins and healthy fats, ensures the intake of different nutrients necessary for health. Choose different colours of foods, vegetables and fruits.

Moderation: Moderation is key to a healthy diet. It involves consuming appropriate portion sizes and limiting intake of foods high in added sugars, saturated fats and sodium.

Nutrient Density: Choosing foods that are nutrient-dense means selecting options that provide a high amount of nutrients relative to their calorie content. Examples include fruits, vegetables, whole grains, lean proteins and low-fat dairy products.

Hydration: Staying hydrated is essential for overall health. Water is the best choice for hydration, but other fluids such as herbal teas and low-fat milk can also contribute to fluid intake.

The following are excerpts from 'Dietary Guidelines for Indians' (as published by Indian Council of Medical Research [ICMR] and National Institute of Nutrition) regarding principles of healthy diets:

> A balanced diet/nutritionally adequate diet should be consumed through a wise choice of food items from a variety of food groups. A healthy meal includes generous amounts of vegetables, adequate whole grains and pulses or beans (*phaliyan*), along with modest portions of nuts and seeds complemented by a selection of fruits and plain fermented yoghurt or curd (*dahi*). It is free of added sugars or contains very minimal amounts and is seasoned with minimal oils/fats and salt for taste.[4]

2

Basics of Diets

Diets are most simple to understand and, at the same time, very difficult to learn and follow. While the basic components of diets (as given in Table 2.1) have been known for several decades, the scientific and general opinions regarding these keep changing. Scientific findings differ because of different methods of assessment of diets, heterogeneity of studies and the variation in the response of different populations to similar diets.

No single diet fits all. The metabolism of each person is different, and so is the digestion. Genes clearly influence how diets affect our bodies.

These days, because of rapid information transfer through social media, unsubstantiated 'claims' regarding diets abound. There are numerous 'designer' diets in other countries and India. For example, for the control of diabetes, one need not undergo extreme diets (such as 'zero carbohydrate diet' or 'blood group diet'), which have little scientific rationale and may harm organ systems. These are often recommended by 'popular' or even 'celebrity' dieticians.

For the formulation of the correct diet beneficial for health, scientific evidence must be followed, and the combined wisdom of physicians and nutritionists is required. Having said that, readers can have a fair idea as to what to eat or what to avoid if they have the scientific knowledge of foods. It is easy to say that this food is harmful and that is good, but most of these opinions are based not on facts but on anecdotal experiences and hearsay.

To know your diets, you need to understand:

1. What are the food groups?
2. What is the science behind various foods?
3. What is the prevalent opinion of experts that is based on evidence?
4. What are the new dietary trends based on clinical studies?

Basic Tools of Dietary Assessment

Abbreviations for Measurement Equivalents

1. Tsp: Teaspoon = 5 ml
2. Tbsp: Tablespoon = 15 ml
3. 1 *katori* (small bowl) = 100 g
4. 1 glass = 250 ml
5. Pcs: pieces
6. 1 Kcal = Cal (calorie)

What Is Glycaemic Index?

1. Glycaemic index (GI) measures carbohydrate quality, that is, how much a carbohydrate will affect blood sugar.
2. It is a ranking of foods from 0 to 100 that tells us whether a carbohydrate food will raise blood sugar (glucose) levels dramatically, moderately or just a little.
3. Carbohydrates with a low glycaemic load value (55 or less) are more slowly digested, absorbed and metabolised and cause a lower and slower rise in blood glucose.
4. Categories:

Low	Intermediate	High
0–55	56–69	more than or equal to 70

What Is Glycaemic Load?

Glycaemic load (GL) is the amount of carbohydrate consumed multiplied by the food's GI, divided by 100. This accounts for both the quality (GI) and quantity (grams of carbohydrates) of the food, providing a more practical measure of blood glucose impact than GI alone. It is categorised as:

Low	Intermediate	High
0–10	11–19	more than or equal to 20

Food Groups

There are only three food groups (macronutrients) that constitute your diet. The calories from each must add up to 100 percent. For example, a typical Indian diet may have the following proportion of food groups: carbohydrates, most common, about 55–60 percent, fats 25–30 percent and proteins 10–15 percent. It must be understood that if we take more carbohydrates within a diet, the intake of other food groups goes down. For example, if a person takes 70 percent carbohydrates, proportionally, the intake of fats and protein combined would be 30 percent. Therefore, the change in proportion of one macronutrient affects others and hence the response to foods (Table 2.1).

TABLE 2.1 Various Food Groups

Food Groups	Examples	Nutrient Value
Carbohydrate	Complex carbohydrates • Brown rice • Whole-wheat flour (*atta*) • Millets (*jowar, bajra*) • Whole wheat (*gehu*) • Barley (*jau*) • Brown rice • Oatmeal • Shredded wheat	• 1 whole-wheat flatbread (*chapati*), 75 Cal • 3 tsp oatmeal (*jai*), ~55 Cal • 3 tsp barley (*jau*), ~50–55 Cal
	Refined carbohydrates • Refined wheat flour (*maida*) • Semolina (*suji*) • White bread • White rice • Soda and sugary drinks • Candies and cookies	• 1 leavened flatbread (*naan*) (100 g), 270 Cal • 1 pc semolina rusk, 43 Cal • 1 slice white bread (25 g), ~65–70 Cal
Proteins	Animal proteins • Poultry • Egg • Fish • Meat • Milk • Curd (*dahi*) • Cottage cheese (*paneer*)	• 1 glass milk (250 ml), 8 g protein • 5 pcs cottage cheese made from cow's milk (40 g), 8 g protein • 1 cooked omelette, • 6.4 g protein • 1 *katori* curd (*dahi*) (100 g), 3.1 g protein
	Plant proteins • Beans such as soybean, kidney beans (*rajma*) • Nuts such as almonds (*badam*), walnuts (*akhrot*) • Chickpeas (*chole*) • Lentils (*dal*) • Spinach (*paalak*) • Tofu	• 1 *katori* chickpeas (*chole*) cooked, ~8–9 g protein • 1 *katori* pea and cottage cheese curry (*matar paneer*), ~7–8 g protein • 1 *katori* spinach greens (*paalak saag*), ~3 g protein

Food Groups	Examples	Nutrient Value
Fats	Saturated fats • Clarified butter (*ghee*) • Butter (*makhan*) • Cream • Coconut oil • Meat • Palm oil	• 1 deep-fried leavened bread (*bhatura*), 2 g saturated fat • 1 *samosa*, 3.9 g saturated fat • 1 deep-fried stuffed pastry (*kachori*), 10 g saturated fat • Depending on cut: meat, 6–10 g saturated fat
	Monounsaturated fatty acids (MUFAs) • Olive oil • Canola oil • Mustard/rapeseed oil • Nuts like almonds (*badam*) • Avocados (*makhanphal*)	• Olive oil, 75% MUFA • Canola, 62% MUFA • Almonds (28 g), 9 g MUFA
	Polyunsaturated fatty acids (PUFAs) *n-3 PUFAs (omega-3 PUFAs)* • Fatty fish such as salmon • Flaxseed oil (*alsi*) • Mustard oil (*sarson ka tel*) • Canola oil • Soybean oil	• Flaxseed (*alsi*) oil, 53% omega-3 PUFAs • Mustard oil (*sarson ka tel*), 14% omega-3 PUFAs
	n-6 PUFAs (omega-6 PUFAs) • Safflower oil • Sunflower oil • Soybean oil • Corn oil • Nuts like almonds	• Safflower oil, 75% omega-6 PUFAs • Sunflower oil, 62% omega-6 PUFAs • Almonds (100 g), 11–12 g omega-6 PUFAs
	Trans fats • *Vanaspati* (partially hydrogenated vegetable oil)	• *Vanaspati* contains about 50% trans-fat (recent regulations have lowered it).
Fibre (part of carbohydrates)	Soluble fibre • Oat bran • Flaxseeds (*alsi*) • Barley (*jau*) • Psyllium husk (*isabghol*)	• 1 avocado, 2.1 g • 1 pear, 1.1–1.5 g • Psyllium husk, 3.5 g per 1 tbsp

Food Groups	Examples	Nutrient Value
		• Cooked oat bran cereal, 3 g per 100 g • Flaxseeds, 1.1 g per 1 tbsp
	Insoluble fibre • Wheat bran (*chokar*) • Rice bran • Whole grains • Fruits like peach, pear • Vegetables like cabbage (*patta gobhi*), spinach (*paalak*)	• 1 slice whole-wheat bread, 1.2 g • 1 *katori* cooked cabbage, 2 g • 1 tbsp flaxseeds, 2.2 g • 1 *katori* cooked brown rice, ~1.4 g

Source: This table has been reproduced from the book *Diabetes with Delight* by Anoop Misra.[1]
Any differences in nutrient values reflect variations in data sources, analytical methods and preparation methods.

Macronutrients

Carbohydrates

1. Carbohydrates are efficiently converted into glucose for energy.
2. They get converted into glucose and affect sugar levels. An appropriate amount of carbohydrates are required for the efficient functioning of the body.
3. The daily carbohydrate intake should be approximately 50–60 percent of total calorie intake for Indians. As 1 g of carbohydrate is equivalent to 4 Cal, a diabetic person on a 1,200 Cal diet should get approximately 600 Cal from carbohydrates (150 g of carbohydrates).
4. Complex carbohydrates should be preferred over products containing refined carbohydrates, for example, whole-grain bread over white (*maida*) bread. Low GI carbohydrate foods like oats (*jai*), unpolished rice, whole pulses, beans (*phaliyan*) and legumes (*sabut dal*) and some whole fruits (cherries, apples [*seb*] and the like) should be preferred.
5. Importantly, the total carbohydrates consumed should be spread throughout the day to ensure that blood sugar levels remain in the desired range. Most people need between two and four complex carb servings (one serving = 15 g of carbohydrate) at a meal for good nutrition. Eating fewer carbs may mean missing out on foods that are important for good health.

Fats

A little amount of fat is needed (essential fatty acids) for the body to function properly. Fat (both visible fat in the form of oil, butter, *ghee* and the like and invisible fat from cereals and pulses) should provide not more than 30 percent of total energy per day. As 1 g of fat is equivalent to 9 Cal, a diabetic person on a 1,200 Cal diet should get approximately 300 Cal from fats (33 g). These calories are stored and used as energy reservoirs. The excess glucose generated from carbs and fats that is not required by the body is stored in the fat cells in the form of triglycerides.

Saturated Fats

It is the kind of fat that mostly comes from animal sources. Saturated fats make the cell membranes stiff and raise cholesterol and blood pressure levels. They are associated with the development of type 2 diabetes, coronary heart diseases and fatty liver. Eating excess saturated fat increases obesity and cholesterol levels. For example, red meat, full-fat dairy products, *ghee*, butter and coconut oils are major sources of saturated fats, which should be avoided.

Unsaturated Fats

The categories of unsaturated fats are:

1. Trans-fats

   Some fats are very bad for health. Trans-fats, which are found in food that has been deep-fried in oils such as *vanaspati*, French fries (*tale hue aaloo*; cooked in such oils) and commercially baked foods are very similar to saturated fats in their physical structure and in their bad effects on cholesterol levels, blood pressure and blood glucose control. Heating and reheating of any oil will generate trans-fats. For example, frying and refrying in the same oil gives rise to trans-fats and needs to be avoided.

2. Monounsaturated fats

   Monounsaturated fats are probably the healthiest type of fat. Olive, canola and mustard oils (*sarson ka tel*) are good sources. The oil in nuts such as almonds (*badam*), pistachios (*pista*), olives and peanuts (*moongphali*) is predominantly monounsaturated fat (Table 2.1).

3. Polyunsaturated fats
   Polyunsaturated fats include omega-3 (n-3 PUFAs) and omega-6 polyunsaturated (n-6 PUFAs), which make the cell membranes more flexible, lower blood pressure and triglycerides, and reduce problems associated with heart disease. Importantly, human beings are unable to make these fatty acids within their bodies. Coldwater fish such as salmon are a rich source of omega-3 PUFAs. In addition, flaxseeds (*alsi*), chia seeds and fish oils contain good amount of omega-3 PUFAs. Omega-6 PUFAs are obtained from corn oil and safflower oil as well as meat obtained from animals that have been fattened on grains (Table 2.1).

Proteins

1. The body uses protein to build, maintain and repair tissues.
2. The protein content of various foods is given in Table 2.2.
3. All individuals need a normal amount of protein.
4. Importantly, low blood protein levels decrease resistance to infections and may even disturb organ functions.
5. The proteins should be of high biological value and provide about 15–20 percent of the calories in the diet, but their quality and quantity will depend upon the blood levels of proteins (serum albumin) and kidney functions. Unfortunately, the intake of dietary protein in Indians is less.

Usually, about 0.8 g/kg protein is required for normal adults. Those who are older adults and have major muscle loss (sarcopenia) will require higher protein in food (up to 1.2–1.5 g/kg), sometimes as supplements.

TABLE 2.2 Protein Content of Various Food Items

Food Category	High Protein	g/ 100gm	Moderate Protein	g/ 100gm	Low Protein	g/ 100gm
Pulses and legumes	Soybean	36–40				
	Whole Bengal gram (*chana dal*)	20–22				
	Black gram dal (*urad dal*)	23				
	Red gram dal (*arhar*)	21				

Food Category	High Protein	g/ 100gm	Moderate Protein	g/ 100gm	Low Protein	g/ 100gm
	Cowpea (*lobia*)	24				
	Whole green gram (*moong dal*)	22				
	Whole horse gram (*kulathi*)	21.7				
	Moth beans (*moth*)	23				
	Kidney beans (*rajma*)	23				
Cereal grains and products			Whole-wheat flour	~11–12	Rice flakes	~6–7
	Chickpea flour (*besan*)	22	Refined wheat flour	10	Puffed rice	~6–7
			Wheat semolina (*suji*)	11	Raw rice	6.8
			Pearl millet (*bajra*)	~10–11	Finger millet (*ragi*)	~7
			Wheat bread	~11–12		
Nuts and oil seeds	Almonds (*badam*)	21				
	Cashew nut (*kaju*)	18				
	Gingelly seeds (*til*)	~18–20				
	Groundnut (*moongphali*)	~25–26				
	Linseed/flaxseed (*alsi*)	~18–19				
	Pistachio nut (*pista*)	20				
	Walnuts (*akhrot*)	15				
Fish and seafood	Herring	20.3				
	Hilsa	21.8				
	Mackerel	21.5				
	Sardine	~20–25				
	Prawns	19.1				
	Rohu	19.7				
	Shrimps	~20–24				
	Surami	19.9				
	Salmon	20.9				
	Tuna	24.5				
Meat and poultry	Mutton	~20–25	Egg, hen (100 g whole) (2 large eggs: 100 g)	~12–13		

Food Category	High Protein	g/ 100gm	Moderate Protein	g/ 100gm	Low Protein	g/ 100gm
	Chicken	~20–23	Egg, white (100 g)	~11		
Milk and milk products	Cow's milk (*chenna*)	18			Cow's milk (full fat)	~3.3–3.5
	Cheese (regular cow's milk cheese)	24			Curd (*dahi*) (cow's milk)	3.1
	Skimmed milk powder	38			Buttermilk (*chaach*)	1
	Cottage cheese (*paneer*, cow's milk)	18			Skimmed milk	2.5
			Tofu	8	Soy milk	~3.3–3.5

Sources: Adapted with data from Longvah *et al.*[2] and United States Department of Agriculture.[3]
Any differences in nutrient values reflect variations in data sources, analytical methods and preparation methods.

Easy Reading 1
Should I Take Protein Supplements?

When people ask me, 'Which protein supplement should I take?', my response is typically straightforward: 'If you're consuming a balanced diet, you likely don't need any.' This advice, however, may not apply to everyone. Those aiming to build significant muscle mass, athletes engaged in intense training or frail and older individuals might benefit from additional protein intake.

Protein supplements have surged in popularity, offering a convenient way to boost protein consumption for various health and fitness goals. Their primary advantage lies in their ease of use, providing a quick protein source without the need for meal preparation. This convenience is particularly appealing to athletes, bodybuilders and individuals with busy lifestyles. These supplements can aid in muscle growth and repair, especially when consumed post-workout. They may also contribute to weight management by promoting satiety and potentially enhancing metabolism. For those with increased protein needs, such as vegetarians, vegans or older adults, these supplements can help fill nutritional gaps.

However, protein supplements are not without their drawbacks. Many commercial products contain added sugars, artificial sweeteners or other additives that may conflict with clean eating objectives. There is also a risk of contamination with heavy metals or other harmful substances in some lower-quality supplements. Excessive consumption can lead to digestive issues such as bloating, gas or constipation. Moreover, over-reliance on supplements may cause individuals to neglect whole food protein sources, which offer a broader range of nutrients and fibre.

Excessive protein intake, particularly from supplements, may have concerning effects on cardiovascular health and other bodily systems. Some studies have associated high-protein diets, especially those rich in animal proteins, with an increased risk of heart disease. This may be due to the higher intake of saturated fats and cholesterol often accompanying animal-based protein sources. Additionally, excessive protein consumption can strain the kidneys, as they must work harder to process and excrete protein metabolism waste products. This is particularly concerning for individuals with pre-existing kidney disease. Some evidence also suggests that very high protein intake might affect bone health by increasing calcium excretion, though this remains a topic of scientific debate. Furthermore, certain protein supplements, particularly those containing added creatine, may cause water retention, potentially leading to temporary increases in blood pressure.

Notably, many individuals can meet their protein needs through a balanced diet alone, making supplements unnecessary and potentially an added expense. As with any significant dietary change, it's advisable to consult with a healthcare professional before incorporating protein supplements into one's routine.

Guidelines for Protein Supplements

According to the 2024 dietary guidelines for Indians, protein supplements are defined as products designed to provide additional dietary protein, often in the form of powders, shakes, or bars. Protein powders are either made from eggs, dairy milk or whey or plant sources such as soybean, peas and rice. Protein powders may also contain added sugars, non-caloric sweeteners and additives such as artificial flavouring, and hence it is not advisable to use them on a regular basis. Overconsuming of protein supplements is therefore not advisable.[2 4]

Fibre

1. There are two forms of fibre: soluble and insoluble.
   i. Soluble fibre attracts water and turns to gel during digestion, thus slowing digestion. It has been known to lower cholesterol, thus helping to prevent heart disease. Soluble fibre is found in oat bran, barley (*jau*), nuts, seeds, beans (*phaliyan*), lentils, peas and some fruits (apple, guava, etc.) and vegetables.
   ii. Insoluble fibre is found in foods such as wheat bran, vegetables (cabbage, *bhindi*, etc.) and whole grains. Fibre speeds up the passage of foods through the stomach and intestines and adds bulk to the stool.
2. Foods that are rich in fibre reduce the rate of glucose absorption, slow the rise of blood sugar levels, slow stomach emptying and delay intestinal transit time.
3. Foods containing high dietary fibre, such as whole cereals and pulses, vegetables, salads and fruits like guava (*amrood*), gooseberry (*amla*), apple (*seb*), pomegranates (*anar*), peaches (*aadu*) and pears (*nashpati*), should be an important part of a meal plan for diabetes.
4. At least four to five servings per day of fruits and vegetables are recommended, wherever possible with edible peel.
5. At least 25–40 g of fibre is recommended per day (Table 2.3).

TABLE 2.3 Fibre Content of Various Foods

Food Category (Per 100 g = ½ cup)	Fibre		
Cereals	Soluble (g)	Insoluble (g)	Total Fibre (g)
Whole-wheat flour (*atta*)	1.6	9.6 (9.7)	11.3
Finger millet (*ragi*)	1.6	9.5	11.1
Pearl millet (*bajra*)	2.2 (2.3)	9.1	11.3 (11.4)
Sorghum (*jowar*)	1.7	8.4	10.2
Barley (*jau*)	2	15	17
White rice (*chawal*)	0.9	3.2	4.1
Pulses			
Whole Bengal gram/ Chickpea (*chole*)	2.5	22.7	25.2
Black chickpeas (*kaala chana*)	4.3	7.5	11.9
Green lentils (*moong dal*)	1.6	7.7	9.3
Red lentils (*masoor dal*)	1.8	8.6	10.4
Red gram lentils (*arhar dal*)	2.3	6.8 (6.6)	9.1
Vegetables			
Curry leaves (*kadi patta*)	2.9	13.4	16.3
Brinjal (*baingan*)	1.7	4.6	6.3
Carrot (*gajar*)	1.4	3.0	4.4
Bitter gourd (*karela*)	0.4	1.7	2.1
Cauliflower (*phool gobhi*)	1.1	2.6	3.7
Cabbage (*patta gobhi*)	0.8	2.0	2.8
Spinach (*paalak*)	0.7	1.8	2.5
Bottle gourd (*ghiya/lauki*)	0.3	1.7	2.0 (2.1)
Fruits			
Guava (*amrood*)	1.4	7.1	8.5
Gooseberry (*amla*)	1.5	5.8 (6.2)	7.3 (7.7)
Pear (*nashpati*)	0.3 (0.4)	4.0	4.3 (4.4)
Apple (*seb*)	1.1	1.4	2.5
Plum (*aaloo bukara*)	0.8	1.2	2.0
Papaya (*papita*)	1.0	1.7	2.7 (2.8)
Strawberry (*stroberee*)	0.5	1.5	2

Cereals	Soluble (g)	Insoluble (g)	Total Fibre (g)
Cherry (*cheree*)	0.4	1.6	2
Orange (*santra*)	0.5	0.6 (0.7)	1.1 (1.2)
Watermelon (*tarbooz*)	0.3	0.3	0.6
Nuts and oil seeds			
Chia seeds	6	18	24
Flaxseed (*alsi*)	9	7	16
Mustard seeds (*sarson ke beej*)	3.4	10.2 (10.6)	13.6 (13.1)
Almond (*badam*)	2.5	10.5	13
Walnuts (*akhrot*)	0.6	4.7	5.3

Source: Data from Saboo *et al.*[5]
Any differences in nutrient values reflect variations in data sources, analytical methods and preparation methods.

Salt

1. Salt is an essential ingredient of food that enhances its taste and flavour. Sodium plays an important role in nerve conduction and fluid balance in the body. Maintenance of sodium balance depends on kidney function.
2. Salt intake should be less than 5 g of sodium chloride (or about 2 g sodium; 1 tsp) per day.
3. Excess salt may increase blood pressure and, thus, increase the risk of heart disease in patients with diabetes, while very low salt intake could be harmful unless specified by the physician.
4. As far as sodium content and health risks are concerned, all salts (table salt, black salt [*kala namak*], rock salt [*sendha namak*] etc.) are similar. The type of salt does not make a meaningful difference; what matters is the quantity consumed.

Sources of Salt

Of the salt we require, 75 percent comes from the food we eat, such as cereals, pulses, vegetables, milk, meat and seafood.

Sources of hidden salt are pickles (*achaar*), frozen foods, *papads*, ketchup, soy sauce, chilli sauce, mustard sauce, chips, salted biscuits, cheese, canned items: fish, vegetables, ready-made soups, vegetable juices, etc.

Dietary sugar is discussed in Chapter 5 (Tables 5.12, 5.13).

3

Current Dietary Trends, Diabetes Reversal and Weight Loss Options

Dietary trends change from time to time. Several decades ago, the Atkins diet was the most popular low-carbohydrate eating plan. It was developed in the 1960s by the cardiologist Robert C. Atkins. In these diets, fats and protein from meat, seafood and eggs were allowed to escalate. The premise was that extra meat and oils increased satiety and led to weight loss. These were initial versions of ketogenic diets. Interestingly, we had also researched a vegetarian Atkins diet in Indians and found that it is effective in causing weight loss.

Since then, several diets have been popular, such as vegan diets, paleo diets and zone diets. Each diet has many variations too. Three popular diets as practised in India are described next. Reversal of diabetes with very low-calorie diets has become very popular within a short period of time, and this phenomenon is backed by robust scientific trials.

Ketogenic Diets (Popularly Known as Keto Diets)

1. A ketogenic diet is a low-carbohydrate, high-fat, moderate-protein diet. It was initially developed for management of epilepsy in 1920. From the 1960s onwards, this diet has been used in the treatment of obesity and many other diseases. The Atkins diet, a variant low-carbohydrate diet, includes limited fat but high protein.
2. As the ketogenic diet restricts carbohydrates, there is not enough sugar available for the body to use as fuel. So it resorts to using body fat. The process of breaking down fat is called ketosis. It produces a good fuel source called ketones,

which is utilised by the body. Please note that much higher levels of ketones than those generated by this diet are seen in patients with uncontrolled type 1 diabetes and could be life-threatening.

3. The reduced amount of carbohydrates in the diet helps eliminate spikes in blood sugar, reducing the need for insulin. Sometimes, the decrease in weight and blood sugar levels is remarkable (and may even result in low sugar levels), sometimes leading to decrease in use of diabetes drugs.

Types of Ketogenic Diets

Many versions of ketogenic diets are popular. A classic keto diet contains 70 percent fat (very high), 25 percent protein and 5 percent carbohydrates (very low), whereas a modified keto diet contains 10–15 percent carbohydrates (low), and the rest of the nutrients are modulated accordingly. Most ketogenic plans allow foods high in saturated fats, meats, coconut oil and butter as well as polyunsaturated fats such as nuts, seeds, avocados (*makhanphal*) and plant oils. In general, the ratio of macronutrients in various versions is as follows:

1. Standard ketogenic diet with 5 percent carbs, 75 percent fats and 20 percent proteins
2. Cyclical ketogenic diet with five days standard ketogenic and two days normal/high carbs
3. Targeted ketogenic diet with addition of carbs and physical workouts
4. High-protein ketogenic diet with 5 percent carbs, 60 percent fats and 35 percent proteins

How Do Ketogenic Diets Lead to Weight Loss?

1. Decreased hunger:
   i. Satiating ('stomach-filling') effects of ketone bodies and high fat content
   ii. Increase in appetite-suppressing hormones
2. Increased combustion and loss of calories due to burning of body fat
3. Fat loss due to a decrease in the hormone insulin

Cautions

1. These diets were first tried in epilepsy and similar disorders; in such cases, these are effective.
2. These diets have been tried for the short term and are not scientifically robust at present.[1] The long-term effects are not known.[2] One must note that while these diets work remarkably well on weight over the short term, the results of these diets on weight loss are similar to general low-fat diets when compared after one year.
3. These are complex diets, not a 'do-it-yourself' diet, and must be followed under the observation of physicians and nutritionists.
4. Compliance with these diets is hard because the high-fat components may be difficult to eat regularly.
5. The risks associated with these diets should be known (explained later). Drastic dietary changes should be discussed with the doctor before implementation.
6. Some drugs used in treatment of diabetes like SGLT2 inhibitors (empagliflozin, dapagliflozin, canagliflozin and the like) also raise ketone bodies, which may cause the risk of ketoacidosis.
7. Some recent studies show that 'keto-like' diets may be linked to higher risk of heart disease. However, these findings are preliminary and need to be ascertained.[3 4]

Benefits

The ketogenic diet has a variety of benefits, including the following:

1. Fast way to lose weight
2. Improved sensitivity to insulin in the body
3. Decrease in blood sugar levels, sometimes even leading to stoppage of diabetes drugs and low blood glucose levels
4. Lowering of blood pressure
5. Control of epilepsy with success

There are several other conditions such as acne, cancer, polycystic ovarian disease and several brain diseases, including Alzheimer's disease, that may benefit from these diets, but evidence is limited.

Adverse Effects

1. 'Keto-flu': Slow thinking, dizziness, fatigue, racing heart, insomnia and cravings. This may decrease after some time.
2. Constipation and gastrointestinal discomfort
3. Leg cramps
4. Bad breath
5. Kidney stones
6. Bone loss
7. Nutrient deficiencies[5]
8. Increased bad cholesterol[6]
9. Poor growth in children
10. Possibility of low blood sugar, or hypoglycaemia, from restricting carbs too much
11. Risk of developing diabetic ketoacidosis at high ketone levels
12. Exacerbation of fatty liver (animal studies)
13. Chance of testing false positive in breath alcohol test

Who Should Not Follow Ketogenic Diets?

1. Pregnant women
2. Individuals with body mass index (BMI) less than 18 kg/m^2 (very thin individuals)
3. Patients with a history of diabetic ketoacidosis
4. Patients on any SGLT2 inhibitors (empagliflozin, dapagliflozin, canagliflozin) used in treatment of diabetes
5. Patients with marked fatty liver or pancreatitis (inflammation of pancreas)
6. Patients with advanced kidney, heart or liver failure
7. Patients with very high triglycerides (blood fats)

Patients should interact with their doctors to understand the pros and cons of keto diets. Those with diabetes and heart disease need to be extra careful. They should understand that low-carb keto diets are good options for weight loss over a limited period. They should always consult their physician or cardiologist before starting on such diets. A sample menu is given in Table 3.1.

TABLE 3.1 Sample Menu for a Modified Vegetarian Ketogenic Diet

Meal		Calories (Cal)	Protein (g)	Fat (g)	Carbohydrate (g)
Breakfast	Scrambled cottage cheese (*paneer bhurji*)	350	20	25	10
	Ingredients: 100 g *paneer*, 1 tbsp oil, 1/4 cup chopped onions, 1/4 cup chopped tomatoes (*tamatar*), spices (turmeric, cumin, *garam masala*)				
Lunch	Spinach cottage cheese curry (*paalak paneer*)				
	Ingredients: 150 g *paneer*, 1 cup spinach (*paalak*), 1 tbsp oil, spices (coriander [*dhania*], cumin, turmeric)	400	26	25	8
Snack	Greek yoghurt (*dahi*) with flaxseeds (*alsi*)	150	8	10	7
	Ingredients: 100 g unsweetened Greek yoghurt, 1 tbsp flaxseeds				
Dinner	Cauliflower (*phool gobhi*) rice with stir-fried vegetables				
	Ingredients: 1 cup cauliflower rice, 1 cup mixed stir-fried vegetables (bell peppers [*shimla mirch*], zucchini, broccoli [*brokolee*]), 1 tbsp oil	300	8	20	10
		Total: 1,200	65	22	13

Source: Author's own compilation. This meal plan represents a modified vegetarian ketogenic-style diet. The macronutrient distribution is lower in carbohydrate and higher in fat than standard vegetarian diets but does not meet classical therapeutic ketogenic diet thresholds.

Easy Reading 2
Ketogenic Diets: The Good and the Ugly

I recently saw a twenty-three-year-old obese (weight 92 kg, BMI 33 kg/m^2) woman. She was smiling, and yet, she looked unsettled. She said, 'Doc, I have been on a keto diet for the last two months and have lost 4 kg weight. Yet I feel feverish, fatigued and dizzy and have plenty of cramps and insomnia. My breath smells so bad. I have trouble eating all that high-fat, oil-laced diet daily.'

The story of keto diets started with the Atkins diets, which rapidly gained popularity. Dr Robert C. Atkins' book *Dr Atkins' New Diet Revolution: The High-Calorie Way to Stay Thin Forever* has sold over 12 million copies and remains a bestseller to this day. The predominantly non-vegetarian Western populations loved this diet (greasy ham, bacon and eggs for breakfast, steak with plenty of cheese for lunch and fish, crab and chicken cooked in a whole lot of butter for dinner). This diet leads to rapid weight loss in many individuals. Low carbohydrates (less than 30 g per day, equivalent to about one and a half *roti*s) in the diet leads the body to find alternate routes to energy generation from acidic ketone bodies (hence, the name ketogenic diet). These ketone bodies provide energy efficiently and suppress appetite. Since then, several similar diets have emerged due to two reasons. First, to consistently consume very low carbs and high fat and protein daily is difficult. Hence, the quantity of carbs per day has been increased in the modified diets. Second, it is not possible for vegetarians to eat a diet designed by Atkins. Hence, *ghee*, coconut oil and so on have been added in surplus.

There are several plus points for this diet. Rapid weight loss can be achieved, sometimes more than that seen in usual calorie-restrictive diets. In patients with diabetes, blood sugar levels and sensitivity to insulin improve, and the need for anti-diabetic medications decreases. These diets may help in patients with polycystic ovaries as well by improving the metabolic environment. Interestingly, robust evidence indicates that these diets have been known to decrease seizures in children resistant to high-dose medications. Further, there is persuasive evidence for the effects of these diets on acne. Although tried, there are no clear benefits in cancers, Parkinson's disease and Alzheimer's disease.

However, many scientists are not ready to accept this diet because of uncertainty regarding benefits and harms. There are several known adverse effects as mentioned earlier and some not known or proven. While short-term weight loss is slightly superior to conventional weight loss diets, long-term results are not yet known. In animals, this diet is known to increase the density of fat in the liver (worsens fatty liver), which remains a concern in humans, although there is a shortage of good data. Recent reports show an increase in bad LDL (low-density lipoprotein) cholesterol with these diets, which could adversely impact heart health. Finally, no robust studies are available on Indians, who have a high prevalence of fatty liver disease and elevated LDL cholesterol. Their blood tends to have excessive fats, potentially leading to dense arterial deposits that may contribute to blockages.

Who should not follow ketogenic diets? First, these diets are a no-no in patients with heart failure and heart rhythm irregularities. Second, patients with disturbed functions of the kidney and the liver and a history of pancreatic inflammation (pancreatitis) must avoid them. For diabetic patients, extra precautions are needed when following these diets. Those who have type 1 diabetes or are diabetic and pregnant should not try this diet. Many diabetic patients who are on drugs such as SGLT2 inhibitors (empagliflozin, dapagliflozin and canagliflozin) should be careful since keto diets and these drugs would have an additive effect on ketogenesis, which could reach dangerous levels. Finally, those who are on blood thinners (Vitamin K-dependent anticoagulation) should avoid keto diets.

It looks like keto diets are not a panacea for weight loss and are only somewhat better than conventional weight loss diets in the short term. So low-carbohydrate ketogenic diets are a reasonable option for rapid weight loss in a young obese individual with no organ dysfunction. This diet should be tried for three to six months under the supervision of nutritionists and physicians. Cholesterol and liver profile should be done to check for any extreme responses. Similarly, in a young obese patient who has been recently diagnosed with diabetes (not on SGLT2 inhibitor drugs), this diet is a reasonable option to check surge of sugars or even for reversal of diabetes. Finally, the effect of very low-carb ketogenic diets on longevity is unknown, and the contrary view also exists.

Note: This article, originally featured in *The Indian Express*, has been revised and updated from its initial published version.

Intermittent Fasting (or Time-Restrictive Eating)

1. Fasting is a traditional practice in various religions in India. Over the last decade, scientific interest has emerged regarding intermittent fasting and body weight and its effects on diabetes.
2. This approach is not exactly a diet but the absence of diet intermittently applied in a methodical manner.
3. Unlike religious fasting, intermittent fasting includes a normal diet in non-fasting periods, as opposed to excess feasting (as practised during Ramadan) or intake of different diets (as in Hindu fasts that include specific non-grain diets) in non-fasting periods.
4. Fasting has a strong rationale for improvement of the basic physiology of the body; it decreases oxidative damage and inflammation and protects tissues. In animals, fasting regimens have been shown to prolong life.
5. Summary:
    i. The three main forms of intermittent fasting (alternate day fasting, the 5:2 diet and time-restricted eating) produce mild to moderate weight loss (3–8 percent loss from the baseline) over short durations (eight to twelve weeks).

ii. The degree of weight loss achieved with intermittent fasting is on a par with that achieved with traditional dieting approaches (daily calorie restriction).
iii. The ability of these intermittent fasting protocols to help to manage weight long-term is still poorly understood as the majority of studies to date have run for short durations.
iv. Some studies demonstrate that intermittent fasting improves cardiometabolic risk factors such as blood pressure, levels of LDL cholesterol and triglycerides, insulin resistance and HbA1c (an indicator of average blood sugar over three months), while others show no benefit on these parameters.[7 8 9]
v. A recent study suggests that it may increase the risk of heart attacks.[10] I have summarised these views in my editorial too.[11]
vi. Intermittent fasting is generally safe and produces few gastrointestinal, neurological, hormonal or metabolic adverse effects.
vii. In patients with diabetes, intermittent fasting may produce low sugar and may harm the heart. Proper medical advice is necessary before following this diet.

Types of Intermittent Fasting Protocols

1. Fasting two/three days out of seven days
2. Low-calorie diets two or three days out of seven days
3. Intermittent fasting on the same day, that is, 16 hours of fasting and 8 hours of eating

In some patients with diabetes, fasting in any manner may be problematic. Many categories of patients with diabetes should not fast.

Summary

1. Patients should be careful as a long period of fasting could cause low blood glucose in any person, more so in patients with diabetes on multiple drugs and/or insulin therapy.
2. Like keto diets, people should understand that these diets should be pursued only for a short period of time.
3. Most of the reviews suggest that weight loss with intermittent fasting is similar to calorie-restrictive conventional weight

loss diets.[12 13 14] Others summarise that it decreases weight, blood sugar, cholesterol and blood pressure.[15] As noted earlier, intermittent fasting should be recommended with caution in individuals at risk of cardiovascular disease (heart disease, stroke) as it may potentially increase their risk.[10]

4. Compared to other usual weight loss diets, intermittent fasting may lead to a higher amount of muscle loss. Accordingly, physical activity and resistance training must be maintained during the diet period. A recent review suggests that most people on intermittent fasting maintain lean muscle mass.[16]

Easy Reading 3

Intermittent Fasting: A Blockbuster Diet or Just Another Fad?

When a patient says I am on an intermittent fasting diet regimen, my mind goes to fasting as an ancient religious ritual by wise men of the past and its continuing practice in most religions. I am also reminded of a Hindi movie where the protagonist goes on a punitive thirty-day fast after committing a 'sin'. Religious people remind me that the purpose of fasting is to strengthen the mind, detoxify the body and add years to life. All this looks too good, or maybe only some parts are good.

The fasted state rings physiological alarm bells in the body systems. It sets in motion three important processes: maintenance and repair, consolidating security (stress responses) and switching on the 'survival mode'. The body stops using sugar as fuel and instead starts consuming an acid called 'ketone bodies'. When fasting is intermittent or prolonged but the provision of essential nutrients is ensured, the body systems become better protected and survival is enhanced. Studies in animals show that fasting prolongs life. Indeed, among many potential options, this may be the only way to prolong life.

Animals have a limited lifespan, which, hence, permits survival studies. Such research is impossible to do in humans. Hence, we look towards other benefits that can be studied over a short time, such as weight loss, decrease in blood sugar and so on. These processes have been studied using three fasting regimens:

alternate day fasting, 5:2 fasting (two days fasting in a week) and time-restricted eating (8–18 hours daily fasting, akin to Ramadan fasting). Results are mostly good in human studies. Body weight, body fat, blood pressure and cholesterol decrease. Weight loss over six to twelve months ranges from 3 to 10 percent. Patients with diabetes improve their blood glucose profile. Fat from organs dissolves, thus enabling a better functional state. Finally, there is some experimental data to show that it may increase memory and delay the onset of Alzheimer's disease.[9 17 18]

Some questions arise. Should we leave traditional daily calorie-restrictive eating (eating a low-calorie diet daily without fasting in hours or days) and embrace intermittent fasting as an approach to weight loss and metabolic control? Could these fasting diets be integrated into everybody's lifestyle? These are some of the unknowns that we face. Most studies comparing fasting diets with calorie-restrictive diets are of short duration (three to six months). A few studies of one-year duration show no difference between an intermittent fasting regimen and daily calorie-restrictive diets.[9] Further, people are also not able to follow stricter regimens like alternate day fasting, and many dropouts are seen in studies.

Our sages who practised fasting were very calm, composed and energetic, but that may not always be the case for those following intermittent fasting. Some people develop irritability, mood disorders, dizziness, fatigue and headache, especially during the early days of the diet regimen. Some patients with diabetes may have a surge of blood glucose in a non-fasting period because of unselected and high-calorie consumption ('I can eat whatever I want during the non-fasting period'). Patients with diabetes must also follow caution as they may have low sugar levels (hypoglycaemia), especially during fasting periods, and high sugar during non-fasting periods, thus majorly upsetting metabolic balance. Such ups and downs in blood sugar may weaken organ systems. Another important point: patients with diabetes taking SGLT2 inhibitor drugs (empagliflozin, canagliflozin, and dapagliflozin) may face a particularly hazardous and acutely developing acidic body ailment (ketoacidosis). Once you lose body fat with intermittent fasting, you may lose muscle too and become weaker. Finally, a recent study shows that intermittent fasting may increase death due to heart disease in the long run.[10] Hence, you cannot learn intermittent fasting from the internet and have a go at it. Your hand must be held by nutritionists and physicians when you decide to take this path.

If you want weight loss and good control in diabetes, blood pressure and lipids, traditional daily calorie-restrictive diets and intermittent fasting diets both produce similar results. However, if you want a longer life and to stop memory loss and brain degenerative diseases, intermittent fasting has positive potential, although no long-term human studies are available. So what will it be? Probably, only a few can follow long-term intermittent fasting, and the benefits are still uncertain. A disciplined, consistent low-calorie diet with all meals on time often achieves results equal to or better than intermittent fasting.

Note: This article, originally featured in *The Indian Express*, has been revised and updated from its initial published version.

Mediterranean Diet

What is the Mediterranean Diet?

The Mediterranean diet is a well-established, evidence-based dietary pattern characterised by high consumption of vegetables, fruits, whole grains, legumes, nuts and seeds; olive oil as the principal source of fat; moderate intake of fish and dairy; and limited intake of red and processed meats, refined carbohydrates and sugary foods.

Health Benefits

Strong evidence from large prospective cohort studies and randomised controlled trials shows that this pattern is associated not only with lower cardiovascular mortality but also with reduced incidence of type 2 diabetes, improved lipid profiles, better insulin sensitivity, lower blood pressure and less central adiposity.

Benefits also extend to a lower risk of stroke, certain cancers, cognitive decline and all-cause mortality.

These effects are attributed to the combined influence of dietary fibre, monounsaturated and polyunsaturated fats, polyphenols and other bioactive compounds that reduce oxidative stress and chronic low-grade inflammation, improve endothelial function and favourably modulate metabolic and molecular pathways.

Importantly, the health advantages arise from the overall dietary pattern and food synergy rather than from any single nutrient or component in isolation.

Benefits in the Indian Population

For high-risk populations such as Indians, who develop cardiometabolic diseases at younger ages and lower BMI, such an anti-inflammatory, cardioprotective dietary model is particularly relevant. In the Indian context, Mediterranean principles can be effectively translated using culturally familiar and locally available foods rather than relying strictly on Western ingredients.

An Indian-adapted Mediterranean-style pattern emphasises whole grains such as millets and whole wheat, a variety of *dal*s, beans and legumes, nuts and seeds, abundant seasonal vegetables and fruits, and the use of traditional oils like mustard or groundnut oil alongside limited use of *ghee* and butter. It also incorporates cardioprotective spices such as turmeric, garlic, cumin and coriander, which contribute additional antioxidant and anti-inflammatory potential. Such adaptations preserve the core features of high plant diversity, healthy fats and minimal ultra-processed foods while improving long-term adherence in Indian settings.

Evidence from Indian patients with coronary artery disease supports its role in lowering cardiometabolic risk, underscoring that Mediterranean dietary benefits are achievable within traditional Indian eating patterns and may also help address related conditions such as fatty liver disease and systemic inflammation, which are highly prevalent in this population.

Vegan Diet

1. These diets comprise only plant-based foods. No animal foods, dairy products and eggs are allowed. In addition, several other animal-derived products (honey, albumin, whey, casein and the like) are also not allowed.
2. Mostly vegetables, fruits, nuts, seeds and grains are included in such diets.

3. These are similar to 'plant-based diets' except that they may include animal products, besides eating vegetables and plants. Plant-based diets are mostly synonymous with vegetarian diets.
4. Vegan diets generally include four to five portions of fruits and vegetables, soy, beans (*phaliyan*), pulses, whole-grain carbs, dried fruits, seeds, tofu and plant-based oils.
5. This type of diet is rich in fibre, polyphenols and antioxidant vitamins.

Benefits of a Vegan Diet

1. On the whole, vegan diets are beneficial for the heart and mortality.[19 20]
2. These diets decrease body weight, blood sugar, blood pressure and lipid levels and thus decrease the risk of diabetes and arterial hardening.[19 21]
3. There is some evidence that vegan diets also decrease the risk of cancer.[19 20]

Limitations of a Vegan Diet and Possible Solutions

1. The exclusion of milk and dairy products in these diets may adversely affect bone strength. The risk of osteoporosis (weak bones due to the loss of calcium) and bone fractures is high. To mitigate calcium deficiency in vegan diet followers, finger millet (*ragi*) provides an excellent solution. It is the richest source of calcium. Additional vitamin D supplementation is also required.
2. Other possible deficiencies in such diets include vitamins B_2, Niacin (B_3), B_{12}, D, iodine, zinc, calcium, potassium and selenium.[22] Vegans should eat whole cereals and pulses since the husks of cereal and pulses have a decent vitamin and mineral profile. Fortified foods or supplementation is advisable as and when required.

Diabetes Reversal Diets (and Other Means for Reversal of Type 2 Diabetes)

Type 2 diabetes has long been viewed as an incurable, chronic condition that often requires lifelong management through medication and insulin. Earlier, it was thought that diabetes reversal was impossible except in the early stages, and the patient would have to remain on drugs or insulin for life. Reversal of diabetes was first seen with the use of Mediterranean diets. Although the term 'reversal' of type 2 diabetes is often used to describe the return of blood glucose to near-normal levels through diet, weight loss or lifestyle interventions, many patients experience a resurgence of hyperglycaemia over time. Therefore, in scientific and clinical literature, the preferred term is 'remission', which indicates that diabetes is under control without medication but may relapse if the underlying metabolic risk factors persist. Nevertheless, for consistency and readability, the term 'reversal' is used throughout this menu and discussion.

Current evidence suggests that substantial weight loss in the initial stages of diabetes can reverse diabetes. This can be achieved through following interventions aimed at substantial weight loss:

1. Very low-calorie diets
2. Bariatric surgery
3. Weight loss drugs/injections (semaglutide, tirzepatide and the like) and a combination of diet and physical activity

Who Is an Apt Patient for Reversal of Diabetes?

1. Recently diagnosed individuals with obesity and type 2 diabetes
2. A patient who is totally intent on reversing diabetes as all the options described next are tough

Use of Dietary Restriction or Drugs for Reversal of Diabetes

1. In 2011, in a small study, eleven people with type 2 diabetes drastically reduced their caloric intake for eight weeks (about 800–1,000 Cal/day), thus reversing the course of their condition. This also reset the functioning of insulin-producing cells.[23] A few more studies also showed the same results, but these studies were done under strict supervision.[24] The question was if this could work in a free-living situation.
2. A study published in December 2017 (the Diabetes Remission Clinical Trial [DiRECT]) in *The Lancet* showed for the first time that individuals living in community could reverse diabetes (46 percent of people) by low-calorie diet intervention.[25] Such intervention could work even in those with diabetes duration of up to six years. It also showed

that substantial weight loss is the key. A five-year follow-up showed that almost 27 percent of people who received the initial intervention were still in remission.[26]

3. Overall, significant weight loss is the single most important factor for reversal of diabetes.[27]
   Interventions:
   i. Aim: To help lose about 15 kg weight.
   ii. Phase 1 (twelve to twenty weeks): Follow very low calorie diets with physical exercise for 30 minutes a day.
   iii. Phase 2: Step up calories gradually and increase exercise.
   iv. Maintenance phase: Maintain weight loss and increase physical activity up to 15,000 steps per day.

About 86 percent of those who lost 15 kg or more reversed diabetes. Recent data showed that about one-third of patients had sustained remission at two years.

1. Such low-calorie diets as used in these studies to reverse diabetes should be planned for appropriate patients by a trained nutritionist. This dietary plan should be carried out under close observation by physicians and nutritionists. A sample menu has been given in Table 3.2.
2. Weight loss due to bariatric surgery could reverse diabetes. Similarly, some drugs could also help in reducing weight and may help reverse diabetes (for example, glucagon-like peptide receptor agonists/dual agonists: semaglutide [commonly known as Rybelsus (oral), Ozempic and Wegovy (injectable)], tirzepatide [commonly known as Mounjaro (injectable)], etc.).
3. Recently, some artificial intelligence-based programmes have been used for the reversal of diabetes. However, more data is needed.[28]
4. Overall, there is a robust relation between weight loss and remission of diabetes, irrespective of the means to achieve this weight loss.

Which Patients Are Not Suited for Reversal of Diabetes?

1. People with type 1 diabetes (juvenile diabetes)
2. Very thin/undernourished people whose BMI (body mass index, derived from the formula weight/height^2) is less than 18 kg/m^2
3. People who have had diabetes for more than fifteen to twenty years

4. Pregnant women
5. Patients with advanced dysfunction of organs (for example, heart failure, cirrhosis of the liver, kidney dysfunction)
6. Young children or older people

TABLE 3.2 Sample Menu for Reversal of Type 2 Diabetes (45% Carbohydrates)

Meal	Menu	Calorie (Cal)	Protein (g)	Fat (g)
Early morning	1 cup green tea (no salt, no honey/sugar)			
Breakfast	2 vegetable-stuffed pancakes (*besan cheela*) with 1 glass salted buttermilk (*chaach*) (carrot [*gajar*]/tomato [*tamatar*]/onion [*pyaz*]/coriander leaves [*dhania*]/lemon juice [*nimbu ka ras*])	200–300 100 (*chaach*)	5–10 5	5–10 3
Mid-morning	1 guava (*amrood*)/small apple (*seb*) (150 g)	50–80	–	–
Lunch	1 bowl spinach cottage cheese (*paalak paneer*) 2 *besan roti* 250 g vegetable salad	250–300 200–250 50–100	10–15 5–8 2	15–20 5–8 –
Evening	Tea without sugar, 1 handful roasted chickpeas (*bhuna chana*)	100–150	5–7	3–5
Dinner	Clear mixed vegetable soup (no potato [*aaloo*]), sautéed broccoli (*brokolee*), mushroom, *paneer*	50–100 200–300	2–5 10–15	1–3 10–15
Bedtime snack	1 cup low-fat milk, 8 almonds (*badam*)	50	3	4
		Total calories: 1,280	Total protein: 65 g (20%)	Total fat: 50 g (35%)

Source: Author's own compilation

Easy Reading 4
We Can Reverse Diabetes with Diet (or Can We?)

Recently, a forty-year-old man asked me, 'Doctor, can I reverse (permanently eliminate/cure) diabetes?' I stated, 'Reversal is a definitive word. Let us just stick to remission (normalisation of blood glucose without use of medicines with no guarantee of permanent reversal).' I further told him, 'I will now explain whether or not it can be applied to you.'

A decade earlier, the reversal of diabetes was considered the 'holy grail' of medicine. Physicians dreamt about it but could not achieve it. Behind this failure was inadequate knowledge about the physiology of diabetes. As research progressed, we started getting more insights into the role being played by the liver in generating and sustaining diabetes. When a person eats lots of saturated fats and calories, liver fat cells rapidly increase in numbers, and when the liver is full of fat, it starts to leak creamy substances (known as free fatty acids) into the blood. Such cream has a great tendency to get deposited in muscles, the pancreas and heart arteries. Deposition in the pancreas impairs the functioning of vital insulin-producing cells, thus critically decreasing insulin levels in the body. Blood sugar rises and does not go down easily.

Having learnt of this cascade of events, the next big question was how this creamy layer can be removed from various organs. The simple solution is to take away the hand that feeds the cream! A nice experiment in the United Kingdom in 2011 made it all look so easy and started the ball rolling for 'reversal of diabetes'.[23] Twelve patients with diabetes were given very low-calorie liquid meals (less than half of the calories that we require daily) for eight weeks under controlled conditions. Investigators were immensely surprised when the blood sugar of all patients normalised within a couple of days. Half of the fat and cream from the liver and the pancreas rapidly disappeared in four to six weeks. Patients remained without medications for a short period of time.

An important question was whether such remarkable results could be duplicated in free-living people over a long period of time. A study from the United Kingdom, carried out in patients living in the community, employed the same dietary principles over one year.[25] First, participants were given severely restricted calories for twelve to twenty weeks, followed by food reintroduction and then long-term weight loss maintenance. An interesting observation was that those who lost 10–15 kg weight normalised their blood glucose. Further, in some people, this remission disappeared in about a year, and they were back to a diabetic state. Since then, other experiments (and massive weight loss after bariatric surgery) have supported these observations.

Based on these studies elsewhere, many commercial clinics in India are offering 'reversal of diabetes' to all patients with diabetes. This is an incorrect practice. An apt person for remission of diabetes through diet and lifestyle changes is the one who has been recently diagnosed, is clearly obese, and is willing to follow difficult and rigorous diet and lifestyle practices over long periods. Those with long-standing diabetes, complications of diabetes, type 1 diabetes and pregnant women should not attempt such modalities. Overall, about 10–20 percent of patients with diabetes may be good candidates for remission.

What are the modalities? Diet alone could be used as has been stated. Usually, it is a low-calorie diet in the initial phase of the reversal programme. The primary aim is to lose a considerable amount of weight. Bariatric surgery is a remarkable modality because if patients are chosen carefully, there is an 80–100 percent chance of remission after major weight loss. Currently, with incredible progress in antidiabetic medications, we have drugs and non-insulin injections (semaglutide, tirzepatide) that can produce substantial weight loss and remove fat/cream from organs, thus demonstrating the potential for remission of diabetes.

Science has given us this great research, which must be applied judiciously. Counselling to my patient continues. After evaluating his clinical profile, I considered him to be a correct candidate for attempting remission of diabetes. Then I told him, 'In this remission protocol, the most crucial fact has not yet been written, that your *strong will* to achieve and then maintain this goal is the most important driver.' That, unfortunately, is not the case with many individuals. Such an approach is not sustainable in many Indian patients.

Note: This article, originally featured in *The Indian Express*, has been revised and updated from its initial published version.

Meal Replacement Diets

1. Meal replacement diets are popular and simple approaches to lose weight.[29] Meal replacement formulas are limited-calorie shakes or bars, which contain mostly high protein and balanced nutrient formulas. These are taken instead of a meal. They are available in various flavours.
2. Such a meal replacement strategy has been endorsed by several organisations, including the American Diabetes Association, primarily to lose weight. A recent meta-analysis shows that this strategy results in significant weight loss.[30]
3. Such meal replacement can be partial (only some part of the meal replaced) or total.
4. We carried out a study using high-protein meal replacement (HPMR). In this twelve-week controlled trial, 122 overweight/obese men and women were administered either a HPMR (two meals were replaced) or a controlled diet with equal calories. Intervention with HPMR led to significant weight loss and improvement in obesity measures, glucose, cholesterol and insulin.[31] The meal replacement was done with protein shakes.

High-Protein Complete Vegetarian Diets (Acronym 'PACER' Diet or Vegetarian Atkins Diet)

Diets that are low in carbohydrates, with high fat and proteins, along with a lifestyle of regular exercise, show good potential in reducing body weight and maintaining muscles. Based on this principle, the Atkins diet was developed. The Atkins diets comprise less than 20 g/day of carbohydrates, approximately 100 g of fat and approximately 150 g/day of proteins to be given initially. This translates to 27 percent protein, 5 percent carbohydrates and 68 percent fats. This diet was successful in achieving weight loss. One potential problem with the Atkins diets was its emphasis on animal products (meat, butter, cheese), which may increase blood cholesterol levels. Further, application of such a diet is likely to be poor in India since the population is largely vegetarian.

We must also know that once protein is increased in the diet, it leads to an increase in several key hormones, glucagon-like peptide-1 being one of the most important. These hormones work on a specific brain centre to decrease appetite and increase satiety, which leads to weight loss.

We designed a modified 'Vegetarian Atkins diet' comprising the following (numbers depict percentage energy intake):

1. Carbohydrate: 36.6 percent
2. Protein: 26.9 percent
    i. Vegetable protein (pulses, legumes): 31.3 percent
    ii. Soy protein: 14.8 percent
    iii. Protein from dairy sources (milk and milk products): 27.9 percent
    iv. Protein supplement: 25.9 percent
3. Fats: 36.5 percent
    i. Saturated fat: 17.4 percent
    ii. Monounsaturated fat: 28.6 percent
    iii. Polyunsaturated fat: 19.9 percent

This diet plan represents a modified vegetarian Atkins diet. Carbohydrate intake is moderate (36.6 percent of calories), protein is moderate-high (26.9 percent), with sources from pulses, soy, dairy and supplements, and fat is moderate (36.5 percent), with emphasis on unsaturated fats. It differs from the classical Atkins diet by being vegetarian, lower in total fat and slightly higher in carbohydrates, making it suitable for type 2 diabetes management.

Results with This Diet in Comparison with the Usual Diet

In our study, following this diet over eight weeks leads to decrease in weight, abdominal circumference, blood pressure and fasting blood sugar, insulin and lipid levels. This vegetarian diet is effective for weight loss.[32]

Easy Reading 5

Gluten-Free Diets Are Not Always Good for Health, Contrary to Popular Opinion

A forty-three-year-old obese female patient with multiple problems (skin lesions, fatigue, depression) told me: 'Doc, I have been told to follow gluten-free diets to cure myself of all these problems.' I asked her: 'Did you have any bowel problems?' She said no. My final question was: 'Was any test related to gluten sensitivity done?' Again, she said no. I advised her that this kind of diet has no place in the management of her problems.

Like many diet fads, it is now popular to prescribe a gluten-free diet as a panacea for all ills. Many people try it to become 'healthier'. Plenty of popular attention is given to gluten as a culprit in many ailments. The science, however, points to limited evidence supporting the use of the gluten-free diet beyond its role in managing gluten-related disorders.[33]

What Is Gluten and How Could It Cause Problems?

Gluten is a protein found in wheat (*gehu*), barley (*jau*) and rye. It is also present in many other foods. It helps maintain the shape of the grain. Mostly, it is synonymous with wheat. Besides *roti*s and breads, it is also found in soups, pasta, cereals, sauce and some salad dressings. Oats (*jai*) may be contaminated with gluten when the same processing equipment is used for both. Gluten is broken down in the intestine by protease enzymes. Undigested gluten can be tolerated by most people. When it is not, then disease occurs.

What Are Celiac Disease and Other Gluten-Related Disorders?

In some people, undigested gluten can be problematic. In some, it causes an autoimmune reaction (the body's cells attacking the intestine), which can cause abdominal fullness, flatulence and diarrhoea. Such a disease is called celiac disease (alternative name, gluten enteropathy). When fully advanced, this can result in anaemia, bone thinning and weight loss. Celiac disease tends to run in families. This disease can be identified by the occurrence of symptoms and positivity of antibodies (Tissue Transglutaminase IgA). Overall, it affects ~1 percent of the population. Avoiding gluten in the diet removes all symptoms.

In some people, gluten sensitivity can cause skin blisters (dermatitis herpetiformis). In other people, symptoms are present after gluten ingestion, but antibodies are absent. These people do not have celiac disease but are termed as gluten-intolerant (non-celiac disease gluten sensitivity). A small number of patients may have gait (walk) disturbances related to gluten. Avoidance of gluten in the diets of these individuals also helps them recover.

The link between modern wheat's higher gluten content and increased immunogenicity is not conclusive. While breeding for elevated gluten may enhance immune responses in some, its direct role in rising gluten sensitivity remains debated due to other contributing factors like diet and genetics. More research is needed for definitive conclusions.

Effect of Gluten-Free Diets in Those Who Do Not Have Celiac Disease or Gluten Intolerance

Long-term gluten intake was not associated with coronary heart disease risk. However, avoiding gluten may reduce whole grain consumption, which could impact cardiovascular health.[34] The findings suggest that gluten-free diets should not be promoted for individuals without celiac disease. Whole grain intake should be emphasised for heart health benefits. A review of large data suggests that, for most healthy people, cutting out gluten from their diet might not be a good idea as it could mean missing out on protective nutrients and potentially increase their risk of type 2 diabetes.[35] While doubts remain regarding the benefits of gluten-free diets, potential harms remain areas of concern. Gluten-free diets may present side effects, such as poor palatability, high costs and socio-psychological adversities. Moreover, it may induce nutritional deficiency due to a low-quality diet.

People with irritable bowel syndrome (IBS) often follow gluten-free diets. However, a recent trial showed that patients with IBS who believed they were gluten-sensitive reacted similarly to wheat, gluten and placebo (sham), suggesting that expectations, rather than gluten itself, may drive symptoms in most cases. Importantly, healthy volunteers in controlled studies did not develop significant symptoms after gluten exposure.[36] Interestingly, a gluten-free diet can sometimes trigger or worsen IBS-like symptoms in predisposed individuals. This can happen because some gluten-free foods might still be high in FODMAPs (fermentable oligosaccharides, disaccharides, monosaccharides and polyols – types of carbohydrates that can cause gas and bloating in sensitive guts), or it could be due to other factors like dietary nickel or histamine intolerance. These potential IBS-like issues, often exacerbated by FODMAPs in seemingly 'safe' gluten-free foods, are frequently underestimated.[37] The question arises: Is this diet frequently a fashion statement?

Gluten-Free Diets Remain Popular Despite the Potential to Cause Harm

By now, it has become clear that gluten is a health problem only for those who react negatively to it (gastrointestinal symptoms, skin problems) or test positive for antibodies (celiac disease). Gluten-free products are commercially available and have become widely popular. The gluten-free food industry has grown majorly in recent times. Many people who are proponents of gluten-free diets for dietary management of various diseases readily prescribe these. Interestingly, some data shows that people who do not have celiac disease are the largest purchasers of gluten-free products.

Reassuringly, most Indians have eaten gluten most of their lives without any adverse side effects, that too for centuries. Following a gluten-free diet may lead to poorer nutrition. Some of these gluten-free foods also have higher fat and sugar content than gluten-containing diets and thus may be unhealthy. Overall, macro- and micronutrient deficiencies may occur due to prolonged use of these diets. Finally, these processed gluten-free products are costly.[38] Gluten-free diets have the potential to do more harm than good in individuals without gluten sensitivity.

Chapatis Are Good Sources of Fibre and Protein. Do Not Stop Eating Them!

Chapatis/rotis, the main source of gluten in Indian diets, are an integral part of meals for most Indians, especially in North India. One medium-sized *roti* has about 3 g fibre and 3.8 g protein. If a person eats four such *rotis* a day, he/she will have eaten 12 g fibre (about one-third of the total daily requirement) and 15 g protein (26 percent of the daily protein requirement). Fibre and protein are important for Indians to decrease risk of heart disease and avoid weakening of muscles/bones. Further, a good amount of fibre helps in lowering cholesterol and betterment of intestinal health.

A physician consultation will tell you if you have celiac disease or gluten intolerance. In 99 percent of the people who do not have these problems, prescribing gluten-free diets for some obscure health reason is incorrect, may be harmful to health and will weigh heavily on the pocket.

Note: This article, originally featured in *The Indian Express*, has been revised and updated from its initial published version.

Easy Reading 6
I Want to Increase My Lifespan!

A sixty-nine-year-old patient asked me, 'Doc, I want to live more. How can I add years to my life? I want my life to be long, useful and not dependent on others.' A fair question. However, the answer is not easy.

Take the inhabitants of Okinawa (a small island south of Japan), a place known for many people living up to 100 years and more. You will find a Japanese inscription on a small plaque in the village of Ogimi there: 'At 80, you are merely a youth. At 90, if your ancestors invite you into heaven, ask them to wait until you are 100—then, you might consider it.'[39] The global debate on increasing longevity invariably centres on the inhabitants of this island. Okinawans eat fewer calories (much comes from sweet potatoes [*shakarakand*]) and consume plenty of vegetables, including bitter melon. They eat seaweed and spices such as turmeric, like in India. Interestingly, the diet contains ten parts carbohydrates and one part protein (Okinawan ratio), unlike most of the currently trending diets. A tight social fabric and a relatively hassle-free active life helps. The genetic make-up of individuals also contributes fewer bad genes (*APOE4*) and plenty of metabolism-friendly genes (*FOXO3*). In a nutshell, this is how we can increase our life, but where can we find such clean air, idyllic settings and such genes? Unfortunately, most urban areas in India have an atmosphere contrary to Okinawa and a worsening lifestyle.

It is reasonable to state that Indians have worse metabolism as compared to many other races. Our bodies harbour inflammation ('fire within'), which corrodes the liver, arteries and kidneys. Ageing molecules are activated, which lead to the withering of organs, including the brain. Within these ageing molecules reside rogue ones, which start cancer. One or multiple diseases emerge, which further cut down life years. Diabetes is one of the most important diseases that can decrease life. Our recent research shows that even prediabetes decreases lifespan.

What can we do to avoid deterioration of our cells? If we cannot entirely avoid atmospheric pollution, we should at least quit smoking, including the company of smokers. We should eat fewer calories by about 10 percent (that is what the Okinawa population eats). Green vegetables and fruits intake should increase to five to seven servings daily. Foods should be rich in polyphenol (berries, nuts, flaxseeds [*alsi*]) and carotenoid (avocado [*makhanphal*], spinach [*paalak*], yellow-fleshed veggies). Tree nuts, fish and omega-3 fatty acids may help. Weight must be maintained at low normal ('lean') with little gain over the years as age progresses. Muscles must be made strong by working on resistance exercises (with weights and elastic bands). Activity must be maintained throughout the day and not in short bursts.

An interesting question is often asked: 'If I settle in Okinawa at the age of forty-five, would I have a longer lifespan?' Not likely. Pure seeds (good lifestyle) to nurture cells must be sown in childhood, and the legacy will be a good and long life. Another caveat is that the lifestyle measures that are so suitable to Okinawa residents may be unsuitable for us. Unlike Okinawans, who have high-carbohydrate meals, Indian bodies will respond better to low-carbohydrate, high-protein foods. Tailoring food and exercise to different races and environments must be considered.

What are the parameters that ensure good metabolic health and longevity: fasting blood sugar below 100 mg/dL, blood pressure below 130/80 mmHg, cholesterol below 150 mg/dL, BMI (body mass index, calculated by the formula weight/height^2) below 23, waist circumference below 80 and 90 cm in women and men, respectively, and a normal-sized liver.

Above all, the most important parameter is the fitness of the individual, which can only be measured in advanced laboratories. It is the sum total of nutrition, exercise, weight and robustness of functions of lungs and heart. If you achieve all this, you will lead a healthier life without serious diseases, even if lifespan does not go beyond 100![40 41]

Note: This article, originally featured in *The Indian Express*, has been revised and updated from its initial published version.

Easy Reading 7

Importance of Current Weight Loss Drugs/Injections

Intensive lifestyle interventions for people with obesity are associated with significant improvements in weight, among other parameters, but often, weight loss is not significant and weight regain is frequent. A number of weight loss drugs were banned, and it seemed that we were at the end of the road for any drug therapy for weight loss. Then came a new class of drugs.[42 43]

Despite widespread awareness about healthy diets and the importance of exercise, many individuals fail to achieve significant weight loss due to genetic, hormonal or behavioural challenges. For those who have tried conventional approaches and failed, GLP-1 RA (glucagon-like peptide-1 receptor agonist) drugs like semaglutide (available in India as oral preparation, Rybelsus, and as injectables, Wegovy and Ozympic) and dual GIP/GLP-1 RA (glucose-dependent insulinotropic polypeptide/glucagon-like peptide-1 receptor agonist) drugs like tirzepatide (available in India as Mounjaro) provide a science-backed option to help manage their condition more effectively. These medications work by mimicking natural hormones that regulate appetite and blood sugar, essentially 'tricking' the brain into feeling fuller for longer periods.

Tirzepatide, in particular, has demonstrated substantial weight loss results, with some patients losing over 20 percent of their body weight. This is almost similar to that seen with bariatric surgery. This is particularly beneficial for individuals with obesity-related complications such as diabetes, hypertension and heart disease. These medications promote gradual and sustained weight loss over time, reducing the risk of regaining lost weight when used properly under medical supervision. Although weight regain may occur after the discontinuation of these potent weight-loss medications, appropriate long-term strategies can be developed to mitigate this effect. Beyond weight reduction, these drugs offer additional benefits such as better blood sugar control, lower cholesterol levels, reduced cardiovascular risk and decreased liver fat. Studies suggest they can also slow kidney disease progression and significantly decrease obstructive sleep apnoea, making them a good intervention for multiple health issues.[44 45]

Tirzepatide, the newly introduced GLP-1-based drug, is intended for individuals with a BMI of 30 kg/m^2 or higher or those with a BMI of 27 kg/m^2 who also have weight-related health problems like type 2 diabetes or hypertension. It is available in India, and its weight loss potential appears to be better than other available drugs.[46] It is not meant for cosmetic weight loss but rather for those whose excess weight poses serious health risks. People with severe kidney or liver disease, a history of thyroid cancer or gastrointestinal disorders should avoid it entirely. People on these drugs should be aware of the correct diet to be followed (increased protein) so that muscle loss can be avoided.

These drugs are available in both oral and injectable forms. Anyone thinking of using semaglutide or tirzepatide should do so under strict medical supervision. Side effects such as nausea, vomiting and, in rare cases, pancreatitis can occur. Progress of patients on these drugs must be monitored closely. Since stopping the drug may lead to weight regain, it should be seen as a long-term commitment rather than a quick fix. Finally, many people on these drugs may lose muscle mass, and diet and appropriate exercises are needed to mitigate this.

4

Diets in Various Diseases and Conditions

Although any well-balanced and healthy diet is good enough for the whole body and generally helpful in avoiding or countering any disease, each disease may be prevented or treated better with specific types of diets. For example, hypertension will respond better with salt restrictions. Further, such diets should be combined with good lifestyle, exercise, avoidance of smoking and so on.

In the following pages, we have discussed evidence-based dietary principles for selected diseases.

Diet for Diabetes

The number of people with type 2 diabetes is increasing in India. Current figures indicate that about 20 percent of people above forty-five years of age have type 2 diabetes, more so in urban areas. It is the leading cause of heart attack, stroke, kidney failure and amputation in India.[1] There is no special 'diabetic diet'. All patients with diabetes should eat normal diets with some restrictions, mainly of intake of simple sugars (sugar and dishes/beverages prepared with sugar) and saturated fats (butter [*makhan*], coconut oil and *ghee*; see Table 2.1). They should have increased amounts of beneficial fats and fibre. The following are basic principles. These principles are different in people with type 1 diabetes, where along with low carbohydrates, enough nutrition is needed to allow for proper growth and development.[2 3 4]

Basic Principles

Carbohydrates

1. Carbohydrates should constitute 45 to 60 percent of total calories. The best way to reduce the total calorie intake is

small portion size and the half plate rule. In every meal, one's plate should have 50 percent vegetables. Vegetable salads are a very good option to reduce the total calorie intake and increase satiety at the same time.

2. These should be food sources with a low GI.
3. Soluble and insoluble fibre content should be high.
4. *Rotis* should be mixed with complex carbs (such as *jowar*, *bajra* and *besan*).
5. Polished white rice should be substituted with millets and brown rice.
6. Eating salads, almonds (*badam*) or vegetables 20–30 minutes before meals can also reduce post-meal sugars.

Fats

1. The amount of saturated fats must be restricted to less than 10 percent calories. It should be further restricted (<7 percent) in those with high triglyceride levels in blood ('blood fats') (>400 mg/dL).
2. Increased amounts of monounsaturated fats and polyunsaturated fats (see Table 2.1) should be consumed.
3. Choose appropriate cooking oils (see Chapter 4, subsection 'Edible Oils', Table 5.11).
4. Minimise/eliminate trans-fatty acids.
5. Dietary cholesterol intake should be less than 300 mg/dL.

Proteins

1. Protein intake should be adequate. At least 15 percent or more of daily calorie intake should be from protein (see Table 2.2).
2. Eggs can be eaten (one egg per day is preferred) unless the patient is having high cholesterol or heart failure (see section on 'Dietary Cholesterol').
3. Non-vegetarians should limit red meat consumption and take fish more often.
4. Vegetarians should increase protein in the diets by having two bowls of lentils (*dal*), soy foods (such as soybeans, tofu or soy chunks), one bowl of curd (*dahi*), 500 ml low-fat milk, nuts and seeds (see Table 2.2).

Fruits, Vegetables, Dairy and Other Nutrients

1. Fruits and vegetables should be three to five servings a day. Fruits should be low GI varieties (see Chapter 2).
2. Green leafy vegetables should be preferred.
3. Dairy products should be taken. Fermented foods like curds (*dahi*) should be increased in the diet.
4. Salt should be restricted.

General Instructions

The physician and the nutritionist should work together to individualise diets for diabetes patients, taking into consideration weight, activity profile, age and treatment (drugs/insulin) of patient. For example, very low carbohydrate intake may lead to low sugars in those patients who are on sulphonylurea drugs (glimepiride, gliclazide) or insulin.

Diets for Hypertension and Stroke

1. In a large analysis of 1.7 million Indian adults, the overall prevalence of hypertension was about 23 percent.[5] It is driven by obesity, urbanisation, stress, diabetes and salt intake. It is the leading factor for development of heart attacks and stroke.
2. Diets for hypertension and stroke are similar in some respects. For example, salt reduction is the key that leads to reduction in blood pressure, and that, in turn, will reduce the possibility of a stroke.
3. Other nutrients that can decrease blood pressure are:
   i. nuts such as almonds (*badam*) (within balanced diets, unsalted)[6],
   ii. berries, and
   iii. potassium-rich foods (citrus fruits).

Foods/Other Factors That Can Increase Blood Pressure

1. Foods containing high salt (see Chapter 2, subsection 'Salt')
2. Foods and beverages containing high caffeine
3. High amount of alcohol ('binge drinking')
4. Sugar-sweetened beverages (SSBs)
5. Liquorice (*mulethi*)
6. Chronic smoking/tobacco intake

Some of these factors have been discussed by Adamczak *et al.*[7]

DASH (Dietary Approaches to Stop Hypertension) Diets

1. This widely recognised diet is designed to decrease blood pressure. Over time, research has demonstrated its diverse health benefits, including a reduced risk of chronic diseases and mortality.
2. The core principle of this diet is to limit salt intake.
3. It emphasises a variety of nutrient-rich foods that may help reduce blood pressure, with potassium, calcium and magnesium being particularly important.[8 9]

Benefits of DASH Diets

The following statements are summarised from various references.

1. Good reduction of blood pressure is observed.[10]
2. These diets may also lead to reduction of weight.
3. Decrease in blood sugar in diabetic patients may occur[11], and risk of diabetes may decrease.[12]
4. This diet may also benefit patients with heart disease and stroke.[13]
5. Cognitive (brain) and mental functions may also improve.[14]
6. There is some evidence of benefit in patients with gout and kidney diseases.
7. There is some evidence to suggest prolongation of life and decrease in some cancers.[15]

Components of DASH diets

1. Eat less salt. One tsp of table salt has 2,325 mg of sodium, and this is the limit of consumption of salt in a day. Avoid addition of salt, and decrease salty snacks. Avoid *chutneys*, pickles (*achaar*), *papad*s and chips. Check the salt content of any commercially available foods before buying it.
2. Eat fruits with meals and as snacks. Do not remove peels as much as possible.
3. Have low-fat dairy, yoghurt (*dahi*) and milk. Avoid high-sodium cheese.
4. Include lean meat, fish, poultry and egg in the diet.
5. Edible nuts and seeds such as almonds (*badam*), pistachios (*pista*) and sunflower seeds (*sarson ke beej*) should be consumed (for example, one fistful of nuts). (See Chapter 5, subsection 'Nuts and Dried Fruits', Tables 5.6 and 5.7).

6. Legumes such as kidney beans (*rajma*) and peas should be eaten at least once a day.

Caution

Marked decrease or stopping salt in the diet may be harmful.

Diet for Liver Dysfunction Associated with Obesity and Diabetes

1. The liver is one of the largest organs of the body. The liver may increase in size due to improper diet, lack of physical activity, excessive body weight and alcohol. This increased liver size leads to damaged liver functions, which may further result in stiffness of the liver (best estimated by a test known as fibroscan). Currently, diet and obesity-related liver disease (metabolic dysfunction–associated steatotic liver disease [MASLD]) is the most common form of liver disease globally and highly prevalent in India.[16]
2. Dietary and lifestyle modification helps to bring the liver back to normal size in most people.
3. The diet for liver disease will depend on the severity of liver dysfunction (mild, fatty liver, severe, cirrhosis of liver) and the presence of obesity and co-morbidities (for example, diabetes, heart disease). It should be individualised for each patient in conjunction with the physician and the nutritionist.
4. Most people who do not take alcohol and have liver disease belong to two categories:
   i. Those with non-alcoholic fatty liver disease: Commonly known as fatty liver (MASLD), mostly caused by imbalanced diets and obesity, it surreptitiously progresses to fibrosis (early damage) and cirrhosis (marked damage) of the liver.
   ii. Those with liver damage due to hepatitis viruses.
5. This kind of liver dysfunction is particularly common in the Indian population, according to our research.[16]

Recommended Diet

1. Consume complex carbohydrates such as whole-wheat flour (*atta*), oats (*jai*), sorghum (*jowar*), barley (*jau*), pearl millet

(*bajra*) and quinoa. Cooking methods like boiling, grilling, roasting and steaming should be used. A non-stick cookware is recommended.

2. At least one serving per day of probiotics such as curd (*dahi*) and fermented foods like tofu and sourdough bread is recommended.
3. Consume at least two to four servings (150 g each) of fish such as salmon, mackerel, trout, tuna and katla per week.
4. Flaxseeds (*alsi*) and chia seeds (2 tsp each/day) should be consumed. Take 2 tsp of ground flaxseeds in the early morning. Chia seeds can be incorporated into daily meals like salads, spiced yoghurt sauce (*raita*) and lemon water.
5. Low-fat dairy (double-toned/skimmed milk; *doodh*), low-fat paneer and curd (*dahi*) (two to three servings per day) should be eaten.
6. It is recommended to have 3 tsp of oils such as olive (*jaitoon*), canola and mustard oil (*sarson ka tel*) per person per day.
7. A handful of unsalted nuts (twenty-five kernels of walnuts [*akhrot*], almonds [*badam*], pistachios [*pista*]) twice per day is recommended.
8. Avocado (*makhanphal*) as guacamole can be applied on toast and consumed daily. Avocado can be eaten as a fruit too.
9. Plenty of beans and legumes (*chana, rajma, lobia, masoor dal*, soya) should be consumed at least once per day.
10. Vegetables and fruits should be consumed. Include three servings of vegetables (two servings of green leafy vegetables).
11. Consumption of coffee is beneficial.

Foods/Drinks to Be Avoided

1. Alcohol (to be strictly avoided)
2. Saturated fats such as *ghee*, butter (*makhan*), coconut oil, palm oil and *dalda* (partially hydrogenated vegetable oil)[17]
3. Trans-fats-generating cooking methods like reheating oils to cook food
4. Simple sugars such as sugar, jaggery (*gur*), sugarcane (*ganna*), maple syrup (used in pancakes/desserts), jams, jellies and marmalade
5. High-fructose corn syrup (HFCS; see Chapter 5), used in sweetened breakfast cereals (*anaj*), sweetened aerated drinks,

fruit juices, syrup used on pancakes, canned fruits and the like

6. Sweet bakery items such as cakes, biscuits, sweet breads, cookies and sugar-laden Indian sweets
7. Animal protein (red and processed meat), especially mutton, pork and bacon[18]

Most of the above points have been summarised in a recent review by Misra *et al.*[19]

Diets and Skeletal Muscles

1. Muscle strength and function differ from person to person. It is stronger in males as compared to females and in certain ethnic groups (for example, African Americans). Muscle strength and function decline with age (sarcopenia), some diseases (diabetes, hypothyroidism and so on), smoking, poor diets and some drugs (for example, steroids).[20]
2. Low muscle mass and power is particularly common in Indians, especially in females.[21]
3. Most older adults have low muscle mass and function along with loss of calcium from bones (osteoporosis). This is the cause of imbalance in walking, bone fractures and low lung functions. Good diet and physical activity generally are helpful in preserving muscle functions.

Useful Tips to Improve Muscle Functions

1. Aerobic physical activity (walking, cycling, swimming) should be done. Resistance exercises (use of age-appropriate repetitive weight training) must be done regularly and is important in older adults.
2. Adequate amount of protein in diets is important.[22] In general, vegetarian diets have low-quality protein. Some items that contain the amino acid leucine (or all branched chain amino acids, including isoleucine and valine, which are not made by the body) are particularly good for muscles (see Table 4.1).

3. People with diabetes have weak skeletal muscles and need adequate protein in the diet, provided kidney functions are normal.[23]
4. Other factors that are important for muscle strength and functions:
   i. Iron to maintain good haemoglobin
   ii. Omega-3 PUFAs (fish oils) (see Table 2.1)
   iii. Adequate amount of calcium and vitamin D

TABLE 4.1 Leucine-Rich Foods

Leucine-Rich Food Sources	Leucine Content/ 100 g
Vegetarian Foods	
Soybeans (uncooked)	8.27
Lentils (*dal*) (uncooked)	7.1
Cowpea (*lobia*) (uncooked)	7.96
Peanuts (*moongphali*)	6.4
Almonds (*badam*)	4.02
Chickpeas (*chole*) and Bengal gram (*chana*) (uncooked)	6.9
Flaxseeds (*alsi*) (raw)	1.24
Walnuts (*akhrot*)	6.87
Pumpkin seeds (*kaddu ke beej*)	2.4
Oats (*jai*)	0.5
Whole milk	0.9
Soy milk	0.24
Asparagus (*shatavari*)	0.13
Non-Vegetarian Foods	
Fish (pink salmon, raw)	1.7–1.8
Chicken (raw)	1.6–1.7
Egg yolk (raw)	1.4
Whole egg (raw)	~1.1–1.2
Egg white (raw)	~1.7–1.8

Source: Excerpt from *Diabetes with Delight* by Anoop Misra.[2]
Any differences in nutrient values reflect variations in data sources, analytical methods and preparation methods.

Nutrition and Skin

The skin is the largest organ in the body and is deeply affected by what you eat.[24] The health of the skin is reflected by its brightness, elasticity, surface, pigment disorders and wrinkling. Besides nutrition, skin is affected by several other factors such as ageing, cigarette smoking, harsh weather including indoor or atmospheric pollution, excessive alcohol intake, stress, lack of sleep, thyroid diseases, obesity, polycystic ovarian disease, diabetes, other endocrine diseases and vitamin deficiencies.

The following would work best for maintaining skin health:

1. Proper hydration
2. Avoiding undue exposure to sun and harsh atmosphere
3. Aerobic exercise
4. Intake of carotenoids (carrots [*gajar*], tomatoes [*tamatar*], spinach [*paalak*], sweet potatoes [*shakarakand*], broccoli [*brokolee*]) and carotene (also photoprotective)[25]
5. Lycopene in tomatoes (acts against solar radiation–induced skin damage)
6. Adequate intake of vitamins B_{12} and E, iron, riboflavin, niacin, lycopene and polyphenols[26]
7. Vitamin A (also used for acne, seborrhoea, psoriasis)
8. Zinc (see Chapter 3 and Table 4.3)
9. Essential fatty acids
10. Green tea and coffee[26]
11. Omega-3 PUFAs (see Easy Reading 8 and section on 'Fish') also used for treatment of psoriasis). Krill oil (rich in omega-3 PUFAs) may be useful as oral and topical agents for skin health.[27]
12. Soy protein (see Table 4.1)
13. Yoghurt and curd (*dahi*), buttermilk (*chaach*)[28]
14. Aloe vera, oral or topical[29]

Diet, Lifestyle and Bone Health

1. Bones need to grow from birth to eighteen years. After that, depending on lifestyle and conditions, they are preserved or undergo decay (termed as osteoporosis) due to progressive decline in calcium content. Almost 10 percent of the world's population suffers from osteoporosis, and it is extremely common in women after menopause. Osteoporosis leads to fracture of bones.
2. Osteoporosis is accelerated in individuals with a sedentary lifestyle, obesity, deficient diets, heavy smokers and some diseases.

3. Indians, especially post-menopausal females, have high prevalence of osteoporosis.[30]

The following would work best for maintaining bone health:

1. Calcium (see Table 6.1 for dietary sources of calcium) and vitamin D (mostly obtained from sun exposure) are necessary for bone health.[31]
2. Dairy product consumption, particularly fermented dairy products, is associated with a lower risk of hip fracture, and vegan diets are associated with increased fracture risk.[32]
3. Other dietary factors associated with reduced fracture risk include at least five servings per day of fruits and vegetables, regular tea drinking and other dietary patterns that provide fibres, polyphenols and fermented dairy products.[32]
4. Aerobic and resistance physical exercise builds up bones.
5. Good protein (see Table 4.1) intake is vital.
6. Increased fat intake and processed foods may harm bones.
7. Increased amount of alcohol damages bones, but low to moderate intake may help bones.
8. Other helpful dietary articles are dried plums[33] and berries. Micronutrients such as lycopene, carotenoids, vitamin B_{12}, potassium, magnesium, silicon, boron, vitamin C, copper, zinc and omega-3 PUFAs are also necessary.[34]
9. All these must be combined with exercise and weight training/elastic band exercises, which improve bone strength.

Diet, Lifestyle and Sexual Dysfunction

Many people have sexual dysfunction (males suffer from erectile dysfunction and premature ejaculation, while females struggle with loss of libido). Diseases, psychological factors and drugs affect sexual functions. Common factors are smoking, a sedentary lifestyle, excessive alcohol abuse, diabetes, vascular diseases, obesity and cannabis use, to name a few. These must be corrected.

The following are some dietary tips that may positively affect sexual health:

1. Smoking is directly related to sexual dysfunction.[35]

2. Follow a healthy diet with plenty of green vegetables and fruits, low fats and low calories.[36] High-protein diets may also help.[37]
3. Intake of nuts increases orgasmic function and sexual desire.[38]
4. Intake of flavanones, anthocyanins and flavones (mostly in fruits) is beneficial.[39]
5. In a large study (21,469 men in the Health Professionals Follow-up Study), consumption of vegetables, fruits, nuts, legumes, fish or other sources of long-chain (omega-3 PUFAs) fats, as well as avoidance of red and processed meats, a diet akin to Mediterranean diets (see Chapter 3), was associated with a lower risk of developing erectile dysfunction.[40]
6. Some studies have linked Korean ginseng to improved sexual functions, but this remains unproven.[41]

Diets and Brain Health

Many people and patients ask me, 'Doc, I am going weak in the brain. I can hardly remember what I learnt yesterday.' They ask for my help to enhance their memory and sharpen it. They also ask for supplements. Here is a scientific take on improving brain health. One should be aware that many of the claims of 'brain-enhancing supplements and drugs' are false.

1. A healthy diet, daily exercise, good social interactions and avoidance of smoking and alcohol abuse will always keep the brain 'young'.
2. There is sound evidence that Mediterranean diets (see Chapter 3) improve brain health. In these diets, nuts and olive oils seem to play an important role.[42]
3. Overall, while associations between dietary factors and depression have been extensively studied, none have been rated as high-quality evidence, indicating that future research may significantly alter current conclusions. Nonetheless, a diet rich in fruits, vegetables and overall healthy eating patterns may be beneficial in general.[43]
4. There are certain nutrients that may help.
    i. Omega-3 PUFAs (abundant in fishes) and, for vegetarians, flaxseeds (*alsi*)/chia seeds (see Chapter 5 and Easy Reading 8)
    ii. Berries[44] (see section on Fruits and Berries; also refer to Table 5.5 and Figure 5.2)

iii. Vitamins (see Chapter 6, 'Supplements and Vitamins')
iv. Daily nuts intake, especially walnuts (see Chapter 5, subsection 'Nuts and Dried Fruits' and Table 5.6 and Table 5.7)

5. A multi-modal intervention (healthy diet, exercise, cognitive training, vascular risk monitoring) is needed. A review highlights that diets like Mediterranean, Nordic, DASH, etc. are associated with reduced cognitive decline, and certain micronutrients (B vitamins, iron, polyphenols) are crucial. The authors stress the importance of a 'whole diet' approach and managing cardiometabolic risk factors in middle age to prevent neurodegenerative disorders.[45]
6. Any low volume of water or salt in the body will temporarily affect memory and cognition.
7. Any calorie deprivation (or low sugar levels, hypoglycaemia) will impair brain activity and performance.
8. Consumption of ultra-processed foods does not lead to optimum brain health.

The Truth About Supplements for Brain Health

Many manufacturers make exaggerated claims about supplements, which often contain many vitamins and minerals. In general, most are not needed if a person is eating a healthy diet.

Recommendations from the Global Council on Brain Health:[46]

1. Many such supplements are not controlled because 'the supplement industry is not as well-regulated as the drug industry'. In other words, taking some of these in uncertain amounts could be harmful.
2. In general, there is not enough evidence that multivitamins are beneficial, and certainly, these cannot replace a good healthy diet.
3. Research is not conclusive about vitamin deficiencies leading to poor brain health.
4. Vitamin B_{12} and folate deficiencies may cause dysfunction of skills and memory.

   If a person is likely to have these deficiencies (due to poor nutrition, poor intestinal absorption, critical illness and so on) or blood tests show low levels, then these vitamins should be given. Indians are deficient in vitamin B_{12}

(especially if vegetarian); hence, it is required more in India than elsewhere.

5. Omega-3 PUFAs: Consumption of fatty fish may improve brain functions. In fatty fish, there is good amount of omega-3 PUFAs (docosahexaenoic acid [DHA]; see Chapter 5, Table 5.10, subsection 'Fishes'), which builds up nerves, especially in childhood. Its benefit in brain health is hinted at but not proven.
6. Vitamin D deficiency is widespread in India. Although there is insufficient evidence that it is beneficial to the brain, it must be supplemented if it is deficient.
7. Iron deficiency: Any decrease in haemoglobin (mostly due to iron deficiency) would lead to a decrease in the oxygenation of the brain. This must be corrected.

Easy Reading 8

Omega-3 Polyunsaturated Fatty Acids: Wonderful Supplements for the Heart and Brain?

'Doc, people say that omega-3 PUFAs from fish are important. I am vegetarian. What should I do?' asks a fifty-six-year-old man.

Omega-3 PUFAs (also called 'fish oils', primarily eicosapentaenoic acid and DHA) are dietary fats with beneficial properties for health. The body does not produce these omega-3 PUFAs, and its pure form is obtained from sea fishes (the liver of lean white fish such as cod and halibut, the body of oily fish such as mackerel, menhaden and salmon, and the fat of marine mammals such as seals and whales). Vegetarian sources are few (explained later). (Nutritional aspects of commercially exploited sources of omega-3 PUFAs from plants, microalgae and macroalgae are discussed by Saini *et al.*[47])

Why are omega-3 PUFAs important to humans? To understand this, one must take a look at studies done in extremely cold geographical locations such as Greenland. Interestingly, the 'Eskimo paradox' is seen here: despite eating dietary fat and cholesterol in a very high amount (40 percent of caloric intake), indigenous people in Greenland (Inuit) showed a low incidence of cardiovascular diseases.[48] These fatty acids are important for regulating blood triglyceride levels, maintaining the integrity of the outer wall of cells and helping complex signals inside the cells. In addition, these are important for increasing the plasticity of the walls of the arteries and suppressing inflammation.

Once we talk of omega-3 PUFAs, heart health comes foremost in our minds. These fatty acids can decrease the tendency for clotting and even prevent heart-related death. While shown in many studies, the beneficial effects on the heart and the arteries continue to be debated.[49] Other uses, some of which are not backed up by conclusive data, include those in various illnesses such as joint inflammation (arthritis), brain decline (cognitive slowness, depression), cancers (for example, prostate), irregularities of the heart (atrial fibrillation) and diabetes. One benefit that has recurrently been a topic of research is the good effects of omega-3 PUFAs in the development of the eye and the brain of foetuses.

The benefit of omega-3 PUFAs on blood triglyceride levels has been proven beyond doubt. According to the American Heart Association, consuming 2 to 4 g (considered a high dose, to be taken under medical supervision) of omega-3 PUFAs per day can lower triglycerides by 20 to 40 percent.[50] In medical practice, we use such doses in some patients with uncontrolled triglyceride levels (seen often in Indians) despite application of optimum diet, exercise and other drugs. Recently, an important trial (REDUCE-IT trial) tested the efficacy of a type of omega-3 PUFA (icosapent ethyl ester of the omega-3 fatty acid EPA) in people who had established heart disease and were on powerful cholesterol-lowering drugs called statins and yet had high triglyceride levels. In this trial, icosapent ethyl ester reduced triglyceride levels and, most importantly, reduced the risk of heart attack and stroke by 25 percent and the risk of heart attack–related death by 20 percent. This type of omega-3 PUFA provides hope for further protection of the heart in people suffering from heart ailments treated with statins.

Vegetarian sources of fatty acids, termed as alpha-linolenic acid, must be converted in the human body to (long-chain) omega-3 PUFAs (same pure form as found in fish), but this conversion is poorly achieved. Hence, vegetarians may have low levels of blood omega-3 PUFAs. The following vegetarian food items contain alpha-linolenic acid (listed here from highest to lowest content): flaxseed (*alsi*) oil and flaxseeds; chia seeds; walnuts (*akhrot*) or walnut oil; canola, soybean and mustard oils (*sarson ka tel*); pistachio (*pista*) nuts; pumpkin seeds (*kaddu ke beej*) and almonds (*badam*). Other food items such as purslane (a green leafy vegetable, *kulpha*) and Brussels sprouts also contain omega-3 PUFAs. Interestingly, the genetic modification of some plants (such as flax and Brassica) has led to the manufacturing of oils that contain omega-3 PUFAs without fish odour. People often take cod liver oil (extracted from livers of cod, haddock, halibut, shark, whales and tuna), thinking that it is a good source of omega-3 PUFAs. While it may not contain as many omega-3 PUFAs as other marine sources listed earlier, it is primarily an important source of vitamin A and vitamin D, which can be harmful in excessive amounts.

Omega-3 PUFAs taken as supplements (fish oil capsules containing EPA and DHA) are generally safe and well tolerated, but they may cause some adverse effects in some people, depending upon dose and duration of use. One must consider that these drugs could cause bleeding, especially if a person is on blood thinner medications. In a few people, these could cause abdominal upset. Concerns about heart irregularity (atrial fibrillation) have also been raised.[49] These should be taken under medical supervision.

What do I tell my patients? Non-vegetarians should eat fish at least twice a week, which on average can provide about 250–500 mg of EPA and DHA per day, and vegetarians should incorporate oils, nuts and seeds mentioned here. Capsules of fish oils will be needed in a few people having high blood triglyceride levels. Without doubt, with enhanced levels of omega-3 PUFAs in the blood, triglycerides and metabolic health are sure to be in a better mode.

Note: This article, originally featured in *The Indian Express*, has been revised and updated from its initial published version.

Diets and Immunity

Various diseases (tuberculosis, viral infections and bacterial and fungal infections) occur frequently in people who have subnormal immunity. It may lead to trivial diseases (recurrent skin infections) to severe ones (septicaemia). Many claims are made about 'immunity-boosting' medications and supplements, but the majority of these are unsubstantiated or false.

The status of immunity depends upon several factors.

1. Age affects immunity. It is better for younger people.
2. Diseases such as diabetes lead to suboptimal immunity, especially when uncontrolled.
3. Poor nutrition and frailty also affect immunity negatively.
4. Individuals on immunosuppressant drugs (for example, steroids) are at high risk of infections.

Nutritional Factors Important for Immunity

Although the factors listed here have been researched and found to be of some use, there is no 'magic bullet' as some scientists/nutritionists claim. A healthy diet with plenty of fruits and vegetables and a sufficient amount of aerobic exercise with sunshine exposure boosts immunity.

However, these factors are important to maintain good immunity.

1. Protein: Low blood protein (albumin) causes dysfunction of blood cells that fight infections. Protein levels may be insufficient in vegetarians (see Chapter 2).
2. Zinc: Low zinc levels may impair T-cell-based immunity and wound healing.
3. Vitamin C (discussed after this section)
4. Vitamin D: Low levels may increase chances of lung infections.
5. Iron: A low haemoglobin concentration (and consequently, low iron) may add to the factors listed here.
6. Vitamin E: Deficiency may enhance immune problems.
7. Supplements with fish oils may help in boosting immunity.
8. Other nutrients being researched are probiotics and green tea.

Vitamin C

1. Initially stated to prevent and alleviate common cold, vitamin C has been popularly sold for enhancing immunity for the last six decades. It is commonly prescribed by physicians also. Some studies have shown that supplementation can improve immunity and decrease sepsis (severe infection in the body), but there are no conclusions on this topic yet.
2. The recommended dietary allowances (RDAs) for vitamin C for adults (more than nineteen years old) are 90 mg for males and 75 mg for females. The requirement is increased in smokers.
3. Vitamin C is commonly found in citrus foods (see Table 4.2).
4. If co-ingested with iron, it increases absorption of iron.
5. Some studies have shown benefit in cancer and cataract prevention.[51]
6. Although 'mega doses' of vitamin C (more than 1 to 2 g daily) have been prescribed for prevention of common cold, chronic diseases and even COVID-19, its benefits are unproven, and it may lead to high uric acid, diarrhoea and kidney stones.[52]

TABLE 4.2 Food Sources of Vitamin C

Food	Milligrams (mg) Per Serving
Fruits	
Indian gooseberry (*amla*) (100 g)	252
White guava (*amrood*) (100 g)	214
Kiwifruit (*kiwi*), 1 medium (100 g)	85
Strawberries (*stroberee*) (100 g)	50
Lemon (*nimbu*) (100 g)	53
Sweet lime pulp (*mausambi*) (100 g)	50
Orange (*santra*), 1 medium (100 g)	53
Mango (*aam*) ripe (100 g)	45
Grapefruit (*chakotara*), medium (62 g)	39
Cantaloupe (*kharbooja*), ½ cup (75 g)	29

Food	Milligrams (mg) Per Serving
Vegetables	
Green capsicum/pepper (*hari shimla mirch*) (100 g)	120
Red capsicum/pepper (*lal shimla mirch*) (100 g)	126
Drumstick (*sehjan ki phalli*) (100 g)	120–157
Radish leaves (*mooli ke patte*) (100 g)	109
Mustard leaves (*sarson ke patte*) (100 g)	60
Broccoli (*brokolee*) cooked, ½ cup (75 g)	51
Cauliflower (*phool gobhi*) (100 g)	47
Spinach (*paalak*), ½ cup (75 g)	30
Cabbage (*patta gobhi*), cooked, ½ cup (75 g)	28
Potato (*aaloo*), 1 small (60 g)	26
Tomato (*tamatar*), 1 medium (100 g)	17

Source: Author's own compilation.
Any differences in nutrient values reflect variations in data sources and analytical methods.

Zinc

1. Zinc is a trace element. The human body does not make zinc; hence, it must be taken in the diet.
2. Zinc is involved in genetic and cellular functions, the ageing process, wound healing and skin health.[53 54] It may have a role in eye function too.
3. Deficiency of zinc, though rare, could lead to short stature in children, loss of taste, more chances of infections (particularly viral), delayed wound healing and skin disorders.
4. Other symptoms are loss of appetite, irritability, generalised hair loss, rough and dry skin, slow wound healing, diarrhoea and nausea. Zinc deficiency may become moderate to severe when intestinal absorption is a problem or due to malabsorption syndromes, chronic alcohol intake, chronic kidney failure and chronic debilitating diseases. Many of these issues have been discussed by Chasapis *et al.*[55]
5. In some studies, zinc supplementation has been found to be of use in treating gastroenteritis, especially diarrhoea in children.[56] Other infections such as flu and pneumonia, common cold,

oral mucosal lesions (mucositis) and gum inflammation (gingivitis), anorexia nervosa (eating disorder termed so as it increases appetite), several skin disorders and acrodermatitis enteropathy have all been reported to be associated with zinc deficiency and may improve with zinc supplementation.

6. It has also been tried in age-related degeneration of the eye (macular degeneration).[57]
7. It could have a role in management of diabetes[58] and bone disorders.
8. It could be useful in people having loss of taste.[59]
9. Some effects have been shown in patients with hypertension.[60]
10. It was extensively used during the COVID-19 pandemic, but its usefulness has been questioned.
11. Sources of zinc are shown in Table 4.3.

TABLE 4.3 Food Sources of Zinc

Food	Milligrams (mg) Per Serving
Pumpkin seeds (*kaddu ke beej*), dried, 1 ounce (30 g)	2.2
Flaxseeds (*alsi*) (100 g)	5
Chia seeds (100 g)	3.9
Yoghurt (*dahi*), low-fat, 8 ounces (230 g)	0.5
Cashews (*kaju*), dry-roasted, 1 ounce (30 g)	1.6
Chickpeas (*chole*), cooked, ½ cup (75 g)	1.3
Instant plain oatmeal, 1 packet (28 g)	1.1
Milk, low-fat, 1 cup (150 ml)	0.5
Almonds (*badam*), dry-roasted, 1 ounce (30 g)	0.9
Kidney beans (*rajma*), cooked, ½ cup (75 g)	0.9
Green peas (*matar*), cooked, ½ cup (75 g)	0.5
Breakfast cereal (*anaj*), fortified with 25 percent of the daily value for zinc, 1 serving	2.8
Chicken, cooked skinless, 3 ounces (100 g)	~1.3–1.5
Chicken leg, roasted, 1 leg (100 g)	2.5
Chicken breast, roasted and skin removed, ½ breast (100 g)	1.4

Source: Author's own compilation.
Any differences in nutrient values reflect variations in data sources, analytical methods and preparation methods.

Vitamin E

1. Vitamin E is a fat-soluble vitamin.
2. The RDA is about 15 mg per day in adults. Food sources of vitamin E are given in Table 4.4.
3. Diseases where vitamin E has proven beneficial: Non-alcoholic fatty liver disease/MASLD (fatty liver not occurring due to chronic excessive alcohol intake and associated with obesity). Treatment of 800 mg per day is given for six months.
4. Diseases where vitamin E has been tried with mixed results:
   i. Prevention of heart disease[61], but other research shows no benefit.[62]
   ii. Brain diseases such as Alzheimer's disease.[63]
   iii. Blood vitamin E levels are shown to be associated with decreased risk of some cancers, however, vitamin E may also increase risk of other cancers, for example, bladder cancer (see discussion later).[64]
   iv. Eye diseases such as cataracts[65] and age-related macular degeneration.
   v. Vitamin E supplementation may help prevent pneumonia[66] and enhance wound healing.[67]
   vi. Skin lesions, muscle cramps and menstrual pain[68] (a few studies only).
   vii. Reduced wheezing/asthma in children.[69]
5. It has no effect on nerve damage due to diabetes but may decrease lancinating pain.[70]
6. Adverse effects of vitamin E:
   i. Long-term use of vitamin E in high doses may increase death rates as reported in a study done in 2005, suggesting caution with high-dose supplemental vitamin E rather than that derived from dietary sources.[71]
   ii. In some studies, it was shown to increase the risk of prostate cancer.[72] However, a 2023 major review found consistent evidence linking higher circulating vitamin E levels to the protective effects of vitamin E (various sources) against certain cancers: cervical cancer (dietary vitamin E), oesophageal cancer (dietary vitamin E), cervical intraepithelial neoplasia (dietary vitamin E), pancreatic cancer (total vitamin E intake) and colorectal cancer (circulating α-tocopherol levels).[69]

TABLE 4.4 Food Sources of Vitamin E

Food	Milligrams (mg) Per Serving
Wheat germ oil (*gehu ke ankur*), 1 tbsp (15 ml)	20.3
Pistachio nuts (*pista*), (30 g)	10.1
Almonds (*badam*), dry-roasted, (30 g)	7.7
Sunflower seeds (*sarson ke beej*), dry-roasted, (30 g)	7.4
Sunflower oil (*surajmukhi ka tel*), 1 tbsp (15 ml)	5.6
Safflower seeds (*kusum ke beej*), 1 tbsp (15 ml)	5.2
Safflower oil (*kusum ka tel*), 1 tbsp (15 ml)	4.6
Hazelnuts (*pahadi badam*), dry-roasted, (30 g)	4.3
Peanut butter (*moongphali ka makhan*), 2 tbsp (30 g)	2.9
Peanuts (*moongphali*), dry-roasted, (30 g)	2.2
Avocado (*makhanphal*), (100 g)	2.07
Corn oil (*makki ka tel*), 1 tbsp (15 ml)	1.9
Spinach (*paalak*), boiled, ½ cup (75 g)	1.9
Broccoli (*brokolee*), chopped and boiled, ½ cup (75 g)	1.2
Soybean oil, 1 tbsp (15 ml)	1.1
Kiwifruit (*kiwi*), 1 medium (70 g)	1.1
Mango (*aam*), ½ cup (75 g)	0.7
Tomato (*tamatar*), raw, 1 medium (100 g)	0.7
Spinach (*paalak*), raw, ½ cup (75 g)	0.6

Source: Author's own compilation.
Any differences in nutrient values reflect variations in data sources, analytical methods and preparation methods.

Selenium

1. Selenium is a trace element. It has multiple actions on inflammation, oxidation and immunity.[73]
2. If selenium levels are low in the body, the individual's immune and nerve functions may be compromised.
3. A few studies show that there is no significant impact of selenium supplementation on skeletal muscles, though the only change after selenium supplementation was a small but statistically significant increase of the mean diameter of muscle fibre type 1.[74]
4. If selenium levels are maintained, it may lead to effects against viruses, including influenza viruses and COVID-19.
5. Pork, beef, chicken, fish, shellfish, eggs, beans (*phaliyan*) and nuts contain selenium.

Diets During Viral Epidemics with Special Reference to COVID-19

Previously, we have referred to specific vitamins and minerals that may affect immunity. In the following paragraphs, we discuss food groups that can be practically consumed during a major epidemic. During the COVID-19 pandemic, diet emerged as a major problem. Confinement at home limited physical activity, while many people consumed unbalanced diets, leading to increased obesity and type 2 diabetes

Practical Guidelines to Improve Immunity (Especially During COVID-19/Other Epidemics)

1. Many of the following points have been discussed in detail by Jayawardena *et al.*[75] and Diabetes (India), National Diabetes Obesity and Cholesterol Foundation (NDOC) and Nutrition Expert Group, India[76]. Consumption of the following will be beneficial.
   i. Fruits; vegetables; legumes (for example, lentils, beans [*phaliyan*]); nuts; whole grains such as unprocessed maize, millet, oats (*jai*), wheat and brown rice; starchy tubers or roots such as potato (*aaloo*); and foods from animal sources (fish, eggs, milk, meat)
   ii. Daily: 2 cups of fruit (4 servings), 2.5 cups of vegetables (5 servings), 180 g of grains and 160 g of non-vegetarian foods (fish, lean meats and poultry)
   iii. Raw vegetables and fresh fruits for snacks, rather than foods that are high in sugar, fat or salt
   iv. Foods with probiotics (curds and yoghurt [*dahi*])
   v. Healthier oils with high MUFAs and PUFAs (for example, olive, canola, mustard, soybean and so on) (see Chapter 5, subsection 'Edible oils' and Table 5.11)
2. Adequate energy should be consumed to maintain ideal body weight.
3. Increase hydration, particularly when fever or gastrointestinal upset occurs.
4. Avoid saturated fats (choose healthy oils, Table 5.11), sugar-rich foods (see Table 5.13), processed foods and extreme diets (like ketogenic diets and intermittent fasting; see Chapter 2).

5. Research on the following foods is inadequate or ongoing, but results are mixed:
   i. Fermented foods (for example, curd [*dahi*], lassi, buttermilk [*chaas*] and fermented carrot or beetroot drink [*kanji*])
   ii. Low-purine diets (some seafood, meat, organ-based foods such as liver)
   iii. Selenium[77]
   iv. Fish oils (see Chapter 5 and Easy Reading 8)
   b. Dietary magnesium
   vi. Foods with some antiviral activity such as extract from pomegranate peel[78], honey[79], *Nigella sativa* seeds (*kalaunji*)[80]

Diet for Hospitalised Patients with COVID-19/Other Severe Infections

Note: The following paragraph includes technical terms suited for a nutritionist. It is included here because of the importance of nutrition in these times and for the sake of completion.

1. If the patient is able to take food orally, taking organ functions into consideration, diets outlined in the previous section can be followed.
2. Oral nutritional supplements (ONS) should be used whenever possible to meet the patient's needs when food fortification is not sufficient to reach nutritional goals.
3. In intubated and ventilated patients in the intensive care unit (ICU), enteral nutrition (EN), that is, feeding through intra-gastric tube, should be started.
4. For patients in the ICU who cannot tolerate full-dose EN during the first week in the ICU, initiating parenteral nutrition (PN), that is, feeding through intravenous line, should be weighed on a case-by-case basis. It should not be started until all strategies to maximise EN tolerance have been attempted.
5. At least 400 Cal/day, including 30 g or more of protein/day, shall be provided by ONS and shall be continued for at least one month. Maintaining hygienic feeding practices and dry storage of ONS is crucial. Otherwise, it may lead to diarrhoea.
6. When using enteral formulas:
   i. Energy: intake should be 25–30 Cal/kg/day (feeding speed: 10–20, up to 30 Cal/h).

ii. Protein supplementation should be 1.2–2.0 g/kg/day for severely sick patients. Increase branched-chain amino acids as they are highly beneficial to preserve muscle mass.
iii. Fat: carbohydrate ratio should be between 30:70 with no respiratory deficiency and 50:50 for ventilated patients.

7. Micronutrients should be provided whenever possible through ONS, EN and PN.
8. There is inadequate research about high-dose vitamin C supplementation and fish oils/omega-3 PUFA lipid emulsion.

Nutrition and Cancer

Although many people and websites state that this food or that food prevents cancer, these claims are mostly unproven. What is generally seen is trends towards improvement. One clear trend is that people who are health-conscious, do daily exercise, avoid smoking or major consumption of alcohol and follow healthy diets such as the Mediterranean diet have lower chances of developing cancer. A corollary to these good habits is a lean, non-obese body, which may ward off cancers. About one-third of all cancers are linked to obesity.

Foods That May Prevent Cancer

1. In general, fruit and vegetable intake is associated with less cancer risk in lung cancer and liver cancer.[81] Among the two, vegetable intake has higher protection potential.
2. In breast cancer, a healthy diet (unrefined cereals [*anaj*], vegetables, fruit, nuts, olive oil, less saturated fatty acids and red meat) might improve overall survival after diagnosis.[82]
3. Moderate consumption of milk is associated with lower risk of bladder cancer.[83]
4. Soy consumption has been shown to be less associated with prostate cancer.[84]
5. In general, an inverse association between adherence to a Mediterranean diet and cancer mortality and risk of several cancer types, especially colorectal cancer, has been seen in a meta-analysis.[85] Similarly, olive oil, instead of oils laden with saturated fat, has been shown to decrease cancer risk.[86]
6. Overall increased nut intake is associated with less chances of early death and cancer.[87]

7. Similarly, intake of whole grain and high fibre is associated with decreased risk of death due to cancers, particularly colorectal cancers.[87]
8. Although curcumin has shown anti-tumour effects (colorectal, pancreatic, breast cancer and so on) in experimental studies, clear effects on human beings are yet to be shown.[88]

Foods That May Increase Chances of Cancer

1. A recent meta-analysis provides robust evidence that red and processed meat intake has a strong association with colorectal, colon and rectal cancer risk.[89]
2. Processed foods such as sugary cereals (*anaj*), ready meals and reconstituted meat products increase cancer risk.[90]
3. High intake of milk increases the risk of prostate cancer.[91]
4. Very hot drinks increase the risk of oesophageal cancer.[92]
5. Some artificial sweeteners (especially aspartame and acesulfame-K), which are used in many food and beverage brands worldwide, were associated with an increased risk of cancers.[93]
6. Aflatoxin, a known cancer-producing substance from certain fungi, can contaminate nuts, corn or rice (southern states like Andhra Pradesh, Tamil Nadu and Karnataka and parts of Gujarat and Rajasthan are the most affected).[94]

Nutrition in Patients Post-Surgery or Chemotherapy

1. The post-surgery/chemotherapy and radiotherapy period is often complicated by low appetite, nausea, vomiting (severe with some chemotherapy drugs) and diarrhoea. All these lead to decrease in food intake and absorption.
2. This decrease may quickly cause multiple nutritional deficiencies. The deficiency of protein in the body is particularly damaging. It causes swelling of the body and legs, anaemia, high chances of infections and decreased healing.
3. Protein can be increased in the diet through the oral route (food, supplements), nasogastric route if patient is unable to take orally, and intravenous drip (special intravenous solutions are required).
4. A balanced intake of carbohydrates, fats, vitamins and minerals is required. It is possible to eat such a balanced diet. However, many times, intravenous or nasogastric tube feeding is required.[95]

5

Various Foods, Nutrients, Spices and Sweeteners

Pulses and Legumes

Pulse and legumes are staple diets in India. People in different regions consume different varieties of pulses and legumes (Table 5.1).

Soybean (Glycine max)

The soybean, or soya bean, is a species of legume native to East Asia, widely grown for its edible bean, which has numerous uses. Unfermented soybeans are used to make soy milk, from which tofu is made. Fermented soy foods include soy sauce, fermented bean paste and so on.

Nutrition Facts

1. Raw mature soybean seeds (per 100 g) have 432 Cal energy, 20.9 g carbs (8.1 g fibre), 19.1 g fat, 34 g protein and a good amount of manganese, iron, folic acid and vitamin K (these values may vary depending on the source).
2. Fat-free soybean meal is widely used in animal feed and in many processed food products. Soy protein is comparable in quality to other legume and pulse proteins and, unlike most plant proteins, contains a relatively balanced amino acid profile, making it one of the best plant-based substitutes for animal protein.
3. Soybeans/soy products have the highest amount of isoflavones in the human diet. Isoflavones are a class of phytoestrogens, plant-derived compounds having weak estrogenic activity (oestrogens are female hormones). Unlike human estrogen, their effects are milder and may vary depending on an individual's hormonal status and gut microbiota.

TABLE 5.1 Nutritional Composition of Different Types of Pulses/Legumes Prioritised According to Protein Content

S. No	Pulses	Hindi Name	Energy (Cal)	Protein (g)	Fat (g)	Carbohydrate (g)	Dietary Fibre (g)	Minerals (g)	Iron (mg)	Calcium (mg)
1	Soybean	Soya *vadi*	432	37.8	19.2	12.79	21.55	4.6	10.4	240
2	Soy nuts	*Bhuna* soya	496	38.5	25.4	30.22	17.7	--	3.9	138
3	Lentil	*Masoor dal*	343	22.8	0.6	47.91	16.66	2.1	7.58	69
4	Green gram	*Hari moong dhuli*	348	23.9	1.35	59.9	9.37	3.5	3.9	75
5	Cowpea	*Lobia*	323	24.1	1	54.5	3.8	3.2	8.6	77
6	Green gram (whole)	*Hari moong sabut*	334	22.5	1.14	46.17	17	3.5	4.4	124
7	Black gram	*Urad dal*	347	24	1.4	59.6	0.9	3.2	3.8	154
8	Kidney beans	*Rajma*	346	22.9	1.3	60.6	4.8	3.2	5.1	260
9	Bengal gram (roasted)	*Bhuna chana*	369	18.76	5.2	39.56	25.22	2.5	9.5	58
10	Red gram	*Arhar dal*	335	22.3	1.7	57.6	1.5	3.5	2.7	73
11	Horse gram	*Kulathi dal*	321	22	0.5	57.2	5.3	3.2	6.77	287
12	Bengal gram	*Chane ki dal*	372	20.8	5.6	59.8	1.2	2.7	5.3	56
13	Bengal gram (whole)	*Kaala chana*	360	17.1	5.3	60.9	3.9	3	4.6	202
14	Field bean (dry)	*Vaal*	347	24.9	0.8	60.1	1.4	3.2	2.7	60
15	Green peas (dried)	*Matar*	93	7.2	0.1	15.9	4.0	0.8	1.5	20
16	Green peas (fresh)	*Matar*	70	5.8	0.4	8.1	5.6	--	1.8	30

Note: All values are per 100 g of edible portion.

Source: Author's own compilation based on data from *Gopalan et al.*[1], US Department of Agriculture[2, 3], Food Standards Australia New Zealand[4], Longvah *et al.*[5]

Any differences in nutrient values reflect variations in data sources, analytical methods and preparation methods.

Popular Health-Centric Uses

Soybeans are rich in protein (38–45 percent), making them the most concentrated plant-based protein source. They also provide about 18–20 percent oil, mainly polyunsaturated fatty acids, including omega-3 and omega-6 PUFAs. The intake of soy is associated with modest benefits in lowering LDL cholesterol, supporting bone health and helping reduce some menopause-related symptoms such as hot flashes. Soy has not become widely popular in India, mainly due to traditional dietary habits, taste preferences, limited culinary familiarity and misconceptions about its effects on hormones and thyroid health.

Scientific Studies

1. There is growing evidence that eating traditional soy foods such as tofu may lower the risk of cancers.[6] However, rigorous trials are needed.
2. Soybeans contain isoflavones, genistein and daidzein, which are phytoestrogen compounds that are potentially beneficial factors in cardiovascular diseases.[7] This effect is more robust in post-menopausal women.
3. Soy phytoestrogens adsorbed onto the soy protein may help in reducing serum cholesterol levels.[8]
4. Trials of isoflavones on bone fragility in women have been inconclusive.
5. These phytoestrogens may help in alleviating post-menopausal symptoms (for example, hot flushes).[9]
6. Epidemiological observations and human clinical studies have shown that adding soy to one's diet is associated with lower diabetes risk.[10]
7. This type of high-protein nutrient is good for building up muscle mass and strength.

How Can Soybean Be Used?

One of the major uses of soybeans globally is as livestock feed, predominantly in the form of soybean meal. Soybeans can also be consumed by humans in cooked or sprouted forms. To cook soybeans, first soak them for at least 4 to 5 hours. Common soybean products include soy sauce, soy milk, tofu, soy chunks (textured vegetable protein), soy nuggets, soy flour, tempeh (a traditional Indonesian food made from fermented soybeans), soy lecithin and soybean oil. Soy flour can also be made by roasting the soybean, removing the coat (hull) and grinding it into flour. The soybean is used to make a product called soy nut butter (*makhan*), which is similar in texture to peanut butter (*moongphali ka makhan*). Roasted and ground soybeans can be used as a caffeine-free substitute for coffee.

Grains, Breads and Rice

Whole Grains

Whole grains (*sampoorna anaj*) contain all essential parts and naturally occurring nutrients of the entire grain seed—the bran, germ and endosperm—comprising 100 percent of the original kernel. Even if the grain has been processed (for example, cracked, crushed or rolled), it is still considered whole grain, provided all components remain in the same proportions as in the original grain.

Which Are Whole Grain Foods?

As per the earlier definition[11] [12], the following will qualify as whole grains:

1. Barley (*jau*)
2. Pearl millets (*bajra*), finger millets (*ragi*)
3. Oats (*jai*), including oatmeal
4. Quinoa (same name in Hindi)
5. Buckwheat (*kuttu*)
6. Corn, including whole cornmeal and popcorn
7. Sorghum (also called *milo*; *jawar*)
8. Wheat (*gehu*), including varieties such as spelt, emmer, farro, einkorn, khorasan, durum and forms such as bulgur, cracked wheat and wheat berries
9. Rye (same name in Hindi)
10. Rice, both brown rice and coloured rice

How Much Whole Grain to Take?

Half of the total grain intake should be whole grains.

Scientific Studies

1. Several scientific studies have shown that the more you consume whole grains within a healthy diet programme, the lower the risk of major diseases such as several cancers, type 2 diabetes and cardiovascular diseases.[13] [14] A good amount of fibre and phytochemicals may be behind such good health outcomes. However, some reviews infer that more studies are required to provide conclusions regarding the effects of whole grains on cardiovascular health.
2. Eating whole grains has good effects on body weight.[15]
3. Whole grain consumption regulates bowel movements.

Sprouted Grains

Sprouted grains (*ankurit anaj*) are whole-grain seeds that have started to grow. There have been some reports of increase in nutrients and vitamins in sprouts.[16] It has not been determined whether these grains are better than whole grains for diabetes, high cholesterol and the like.

Breads (Not Including Indian Rotis/Chapatis)

Breads are our daily food. One often tends to confuse the different types of breads and their possible health effects.

1. White bread (one slice, 77 Cal): It is processed to remove bran and the germ from wheat kernels, leaving only the endosperm. The colour is white, but nutrients are few. It is a high GI food.
2. Wheat bread: Wheat bread is made using wheat flour and should not be confused with whole-wheat bread.
3. Whole-wheat bread: This bread contains bran, the germ and the endosperm of the wheat kernel and is nutritionally superior to white bread because it has more fibre, vitamins, minerals and phytochemicals. The GI is often lower than white bread.
4. Whole-grain bread: It is made of whole grains, including whole barley (*jau*), brown rice and whole-grain oats (*jai*). This bread contains more fibre and vitamins. The intake of these breads generally produces a lower post-meal glucose response, although the glycaemic index varies depending on processing and formulation.
5. Multigrain bread: This contains multiple grains, but all of them may not be whole grains, and bran and germ may have

been removed in some/all of them. Labels such as 'refined', 'bleached' or 'enriched wheat flour' indicate that the grain has been processed and does not qualify as a whole grain, even if small amounts of bran are added back.

6. Other mixed breads: These may contain a mixture of other foods, seeds, mushrooms and so on.
7. Sourdough bread: This bread is made by the fermentation of dough using lactobacilli and yeast, thus giving it a sour taste. This fermentation can modify starch structure and slow digestion, and some studies suggest that sourdough bread may produce a lower post-meal glucose and insulin response compared with conventional bread, sometimes even when made from whole-wheat flour.
8. Rye bread: A very popular northern European sandwich called Reuben sandwich is made with rye bread. These are made from crushed or ground whole rye kernels. Rye flour is mixed in different percentages with other flours to give a variety of tastes, colours and textures.
9. Pumpernickel bread: Pumpernickel bread is a German variety of rye bread made using only rye flour and a long baking time set at a low temperature.
10. Baguette: Baguette is a French bread made as long, crusty loaves. It is made of flour, water, yeast and salt. These are famous for their crisp exteriors and soft, chewy interiors.
11. Ciabatta: Panini, the Italian sandwich, is made with ciabatta. Made from a dough that includes olive oil, ciabatta is known for its porous interior with alveolar-like air pockets.

Indian Breads

Difference and GI of some breads is discussed by Gold, Yusof *et al.* and Najjar *et al.*[17] [18] [19]

1. R*otis* (flatbread)
   i. *Chapati* (one *roti*, 40 g, 120 Cal): This is the usual bread consumed by most people in India.
   ii. *Rumali roti* (used mostly in North India): An elongated thin bread, it is made with whole-wheat flour (*atta*) and white wheaten *maida* flour (all-purpose flour) further kneaded with milk and salt.

iii. *Makke ki roti* (used mostly in Punjab, North India): This *roti* is made of maize flour (*makke ka aata*).

iv. *Tandoori roti* (used in North India): This thick *roti* is made with wheat flour and heated in a *tandoor*.

2. *Dosa* (consumed mostly in South India, about 130 Cal in a plain dosa): It is a thin pancake made from a fermented batter of rice and black gram (*urad dal*).
3. *Appam* (eaten in South India): This is made with fermented rice batter and coconut milk.
4. *Bhatura* (eaten in North India, about 85 g per piece, 250 Cal): This is a deep-fried (in *ghee* or oil) bread made of white flour (*maida*).
5. *Cheela* (eaten in North India): These are made of a mixture of flours, usually pulse (*dal*) flour or gram flour (*besan*). Variations include mung beans (*moong dal*), oats or millet (*mota anaj*) flours.
6. *Kachori* (eaten in North India): It is a deep-fried thick bread with various fillings.
7. *Kulcha* (eaten in North India): It is a flatbread made of *maida* flour, water, a pinch of salt and a leavening agent like yeast.
8. *Puran poli:* A popular Maharashtrian delicacy, it is a kind of *paratha* stuffed with *chana dal*, jaggery (*gur*) and coconut mixture and then cooked with some *ghee*.
9. *Puri*: The bread of happy occasions, *puri* is unleavened and made with whole-wheat dough and is deep-fried.
10. *Paratha* (eaten mostly in North India, one average non-stuffed wheat *paratha*, about 120 Cal): A flatbread made of wheat dough and fried on a *tawa* (frying pan), it could be stuffed with tomatoes (*tamatar*), eggs and so on. About thirty types are available.
11. *Naan* (commonly eaten in North India; one average-sized naan contains 200–300 Cal): It is a thick flatbread traditionally made from wheat or refined (*maida*) flour, active dry yeast, salt and water and often includes yoghurt (*dahi*) or milk, a small amount of sugar and oil or ghee to enhance softness and flavour.
12. *Litti* (eaten in North India, Bihar): Whole-wheat flour is mixed with roasted chickpea flour (*sattu*) and a lot of *ghee* and then roasted.
13. *Baati*: Round and small baked dough balls are served with lentils (*dal*) and *choorma* (a traditional Indian sweet made from

coarsely ground whole wheat roasted in *ghee* and mixed with jaggery [*gur*] or sugar, often flavoured with cardamom and garnished with dried fruits).

14. *Sheermaal:* An inseparable part of traditional Awadhi and Nizami cuisine, it is a leavened bread cooked in a tandoor oven. It is flavoured with saffron and has a mildly sweet taste.
15. *Bakarkhani:* It is a leavened bread with a biscuit-like texture. It is mildly spiced, sweet and flavoured with saffron. It is prepared as a part of Eid celebrations and tastes great with meats and gravies.
16 *Pathiri:* A white, thin pancake made with rice flour, *pathiri* is popular with Malabari Muslims and is an essential part of Iftaar during Ramazan.
17. *Thalipeeth:* Popular in Maharashtra, Gujarat and some other parts of western India, it is made with rice, wheat, sorghum (*jowar*), pearl millet (*bajra*), black gram (*urad*) and Bengal gram (*chana*). It is spicy and savoury.
18. *Thepla:* Made with whole-wheat flour, gram flour, fenugreek leaves and spices, this Gujarati bread is soft and has a longer shelf life than most breads.

Wheat

Wheat is a cereal (*anaj*) grain that is staple food worldwide. In India, wheat *roti*s are a staple food, especially in North India.

Nutrition Facts

1. Nutrition facts about wheat as compared to other cereals are given in Table 5.2 (these values may vary depending on the source).
2. While most people know wheat as a source of carbohydrates, it is a good source of protein and fibre, both beneficial to the body.
3. It contains a good amount of vitamins thiamine and niacin.
4. A small part of wheat protein is gluten. Some people (less than 1 percent of the population) have an autoimmune-based (gluten antibodies are present) sensitivity to it. These people develop abdominal bloating and diarrhoea after ingesting gluten. Such symptoms may also occur in some people who do not have antibodies. Gluten-free diets are a current fad, often followed for weight loss and in the hope of improving the status of various diseases (see Easy Reading 5).

Where Is Wheat Used?

Wheat is used in bread, porridge, breakfast cereals (*anaj*), biscuits, pizza, pasta, wheat-based noodles, semolina (*suji*), cakes, wheat rolls, doughnuts, beer, wheat-based vodka and so on.

Other Cereals in India

Like wheat, several other cereals (*anaj*) are consumed in various regions of India. Calorie values and other nutrition facts of various cereals are given in Table 5.2.

Maida flour is commonly used to make *naan, rumali roti*s (see previous discussion on Indian breads), noodles, deep-fried unleavened flatbread (*puri*s), doughnuts, pizzas, momos, crispy semolina or wheat shells filled with tangy spiced water (*panipuri*s) and bread. It is a wheat flour made from endosperm, which is finely milled, refined and bleached (with bleaching agents) without any bran ('refined carbohydrate').

Gram flour (*besan*) is made from Bengal gram (*chana dal*) and contains a high proportion of carbohydrates. It is considered a healthier flour variety, as it is rich in fibre and protein compared to many other flours and does not contain gluten. Besan provides approximately 380 Cal of energy, 20–22 g of protein, 58–60 g of carbohydrate, 10–11 g of dietary fibre and 6–7 g of fat per 100 g. It has low GI value (approximately 27 to 35), making it useful for people with diabetes. *Besan roti* and *cheela* are ideal for a person with type 2 diabetes.

Comments on Table 5.2

1. Overall, whole wheat still compares favourably with other millets, and it is the cheapest.
2. Finger millet (*ragi*) has the lowest calories/100 g weight and the lowest fat content.
3. Pearl millet (*bajra*) and pearl barley (*jau*) have the lowest GI, indicating their usefulness in patients with diabetes and obesity.
4. Pearl barley (*jau*) has the highest fibre.
5. Quinoa has the lowest amount of carbs. Some whole grains such as quinoa can help reduce postprandial glycaemic response due to their lower GI.[21 22]
6. Corn (*bhutta*) and finger millet (*ragi*) have high GI.

TABLE 5.2 Nutritive Value of Uncooked Cereals

Nutritive Values of 100 g of Uncooked Wheat and Other Cereals Commonly Consumed in India

	Whole wheat (*Gehu*, Triticum aestivum)	Sorghum (*Jowar*, Sorghum bicolor)	Finger Millet (*Ragi*, Eleusine coracana)	Pearl Millet (*Bajra*, Pennisetum glaucum)	Corn (*Bhutta*, Zea mays)	Pearl Barley (*Jau*, Hordeum vulgare)	Oats (*Jai*, Avena sativa)	Quinoa (Chenopodium quinoa)
Energy (Cal)	350	349	328	361	365	352	379	360
Macronutrients								
Carbohydrate (g)	71.2	72.6	72	67.5	74.26	77.72	67.70	67.44
Fibre (g)	12.5	9.7	11.5	11.3	7.3	15.6	10.1	7.0
Protein (g)	11.8	10.4	7.3	11.6	9.42	9.91	13.15	12.79
Fat (g)	1.5	1.9	1.3	5.0	4.74	1.16	6.52	5.81
Micronutrients								
Iron (mg)	5.3	4.1	3.9	8.0	2.71	2.5	4.25	8.37
Potassium (mg)	284	131	408	307	287	280	362	-
Calcium (mg)	41	25	344	42	7	29	52	0
GI	91	77	104	55	156	53	65^	63

Source: Author's own compilation. Values given here may vary depending on source. See values of quinoa as given by Nowak *et al.*[20] also.
Any differences in nutrient values reflect variations in data sources, analytical methods and preparation methods.

Overall assessment of GI is based on both regional food studies and international databases.[23 24 25]

Quinoa

1. Quinoa is being increasingly consumed as 'healthy food'.[26] The GI of quinoa ranges from 51.3 to 78.3, with an average of 63.4, and the GL is from 25.6 to 39, with an average of 31.7. Hence, this quinoa variety can be categorised as a medium GI or high GL food.[22]
2. In general, high variations in nutrient contents of quinoa were observed per 100 g of edible portion on fresh weight basis—protein (9.1–15.7 g), total fat (4.0–7.6 g) and dietary fibre (8.8–14.1 g).[20] It contains all nine essential amino acids and has moderate amount of fibre. Please note that variations in these values are considerable depending on the source.
3. Recent research strongly suggests that non-essential nutrients such as phytochemicals of quinoa and amaranth (*rajgeera*) may also have potential beneficial effects for health.[27]
4. Apart from the macronutrients mentioned in Table 5.2, it is rich in folate, iron, magnesium and zinc (these values may vary depending on the source).
5. The calorie content of cooked quinoa is about 120 Cal/100 g. It may have some benefit in patients with diabetes, but more data is needed. Please note that for this issue, pearl millet (*bajra*) and pearl barley (*jau*) may offer comparable or greater metabolic benefits and are often more affordable in Indian settings.
6. It is gluten-free.[26]

Ragi

1. *Ragi* is a popular ingredient in several Indian dishes, particularly in South India.
2. It is rich in iron, calcium and potassium; hence, it may be suitable for aiding growth in children. However, the bioavailability of some minerals, especially iron, may be limited due to naturally occurring phytates.
3. It has low calorie and fat content (see Table 5.2). Hence, it may be beneficial in preventing obesity, although scientific data is lacking (these values may vary depending on the source).

4. The glycaemic response to *ragi* varies with processing. Some reports state that it has high GI and, hence, may not be suitable for people with diabetes.[28]

Oats

These are whole-grain seeds from the oat plant.

Nutrition Facts

1. Per 100 g, oats (*jai*) contain 394 Cal, 66.3 g carbohydrates (10–11 g fibre, beta-glucan, soluble fibre), 11.6 g protein, 7 g fat, a high amount of vitamin K and a good amount of thiamine, vitamin B_6, iron, manganese and zinc (these values may vary depending on the source). The GI of oats can vary depending on factors like processing and cooking methods. Less processed forms such as steel-cut or rolled oats have a lower GI (approximately 45–55), while quick oats and instant oats tend to have a higher GI due to greater processing, increased surface area and faster digestion.
2. Oats are rich in soluble fibre (beta-glucan) and provide a moderate amount of protein (approximately 11–17 g per 100 g dry oats). While they supply several important vitamins and minerals, their protein quality is not equivalent to soy, eggs or meat, as they are relatively low in lysine. In comparison, soybeans contain about 36 g protein per 100 g and are a complete plant protein.
3. Avenalin proteins in oats may rarely cause gluten sensitivity.

Scientific Studies

1. Many studies, including those done in India by us[29], show the effective cholesterol-lowering properties of oats. In our study, patients were served 70 g of oats twice a day in the form of porridge and *upma* (a thick porridge from oats with seasonings and vegetables). It resulted in 8 percent decline in blood cholesterol levels. In a patient with high cholesterol, diabetes and heart disease, such a reduction is significant.
2. There is some evidence that it may reduce weight and blood sugar levels in overweight diabetic patients.[30]
3. Oats are generally safe for gluten-sensitive patients.[31]

4. In protein-deficient people, oats are a good source of protein and should be included in diets.[32]

Millets

Millets are part of the traditional diet of the Indian population. In recent times, it has been given major importance and advertised widely as healthy food by the Indian government. Notably, there are different types of millets, all with different nutritive properties. The type of millet must be carefully chosen to suit the profile of the person consuming it. Some millets have been described in Table 5.3. India has indeed taken steps to popularise millets through campaigns, policies and public awareness programmes, recognising their role in enhancing nutrition, food security and the welfare of farmers. In addition to a plethora of health advantages, they are also beneficial for the environment because they require less water and other resources to grow.

The Government of India requested that the United Nations declare 2023 as the International Year of Millets to raise awareness and increase millets' production and consumption.

What Are Millets?

The major millets are sorghum (*jowar*), pearl (*bajra*) and finger (*ragi*). The minor millets are foxtail (*kangani*), kodo (*kodra*), barnyard (*sanva*), proso (*punarva/chena*), browntop (*murat*), little millet (*saama*), buckwheat (*kuttu*) and amaranth (*rajgeera*). Some commonly used millets have been shown further in Figure 5.1. Barley (*jau*) is a cereal (*anaj*) grain belonging to the grass family. It is not a millet but is included here because of its nutritional properties.

Health Benefits of Millets

1. The low GI of barley (*jau*, 53) and pearl millet (*bajra*, 55) makes them suitable for people with diabetes.
2. Amaranth (*rajgeera*) is a very good source of total protein (13 g/100 g) among all the cereals and millets.
3. Finger millet (*ragi*) is a rich source of calcium (344 mg/100 g). It is good for those suffering from lactose intolerance and helpful in developing strong bones. Since some reports state that it has a slightly higher GI than other millets (depending upon processing), it must be used in combination with other millets, pulses and cereals (see Table 5.2) by people with diabetes.[23]

4. Millets are a good source of dietary fibre (pearl millet [*bajra*] 12 g/100 g, barley [*jau*] 15 g/100 g), which is helpful to reduce the risk of various non-communicable diseases such as obesity, type 2 diabetes, cardiovascular diseases and colon cancer (see Chapter 4).
5. Pearl millet (*bajra*) is a rich source of iron (8 mg/100 g), helpful in treating anaemia.

TABLE 5.3 Commonly Used Millets in India (all values are expressed as g per 100 g)

Name	Calorie	Protein (g)	GI	GL	Available Carbohydrates (g)	Fat (g)
Pearl millet (*bajra*)	348	11	45	12	61.8	5.4
Finger millet (*ragi*)	320	7.2	84	42	66.8	1.9
Foxtail millet (*kangani/kakum*)	349	12.3	55	10–12	60.1	4.3
Sorghum (*jowar*)	334	10	62	12–14	67.7	1.7
Little millet (*samai/kutki*)	346.3	10	64	10–12	65.6	3.9
Barley (*jau*)	315	10.9	37		61.3	1.3

Source: Author's own compilation. Values given here are taken from various sources, including Longvah *et al.*[5] and Foster-Powell *et al.*[33]

Differences in nutrient, GI and GL values for the same millet from Table 5.3 reflect variations in data sources, grain variety, processing, cooking methods and whether total or available carbohydrates are reported. GI is a biological measure rather than a fixed food property.

FIGURE 5.1 Commonly Grown Millets in India

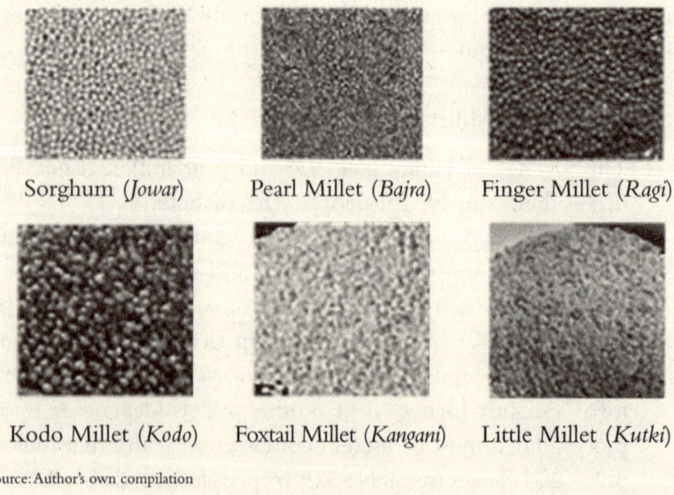

Source: Author's own compilation

Rice

These are the seeds of the grass *Oryza sativa*, commonly known as *chawal* and *bhaat* in India. Rice is perhaps the most common carbohydrate-based food eaten worldwide and is the staple diet in South Asia, China and far eastern countries. The following are the various commonly eaten varieties:

1. White rice: Milled rice (*chamkaya hua chawal*) with husk, bran and germ removed
2. Brown rice: Whole grain with only the inedible hull of the seed removed
3. Germinated rice
4. Glutinous rice
5. Other varieties: Other rice varieties include black, purple and red rice, available in both milled (polished) and whole grain (unpolished) forms

Nutrition Facts

The nutritive value of different types of rice is given in Table 5.4 (these values may vary depending on the source). Brown rice (*bhura chawal,* whole grain) has fibre, and the GI is lower than that of white rice.

Scientific Studies

Several scientific studies exist, mostly pertaining to the effects of rice on blood glucose levels and obesity. The following are conclusions:

1. Brown rice provides more fibre, micronutrients and bioactive compounds than white rice, particularly in germinated or glutinous varieties, which may slow gastric emptying and glucose absorption. It is reported that replacing 50 g/d (cooked, equivalent to one-third serving per day) intake of white rice with the same amount of brown rice was associated with a 16 percent lower risk of type 2 diabetes.[34]
2. Parboiled rice (*sela chawal*) may offer better post-meal sugar control than both white rice and brown rice.[35]
3. Increased ingestion of white rice has also been linked to weight gain and the risk of type 2 diabetes in some studies.

Red Yeast Rice

Red yeast rice (*laal khameer chawal*) contains a fungus (*Monascus purpureus*), which naturally produces monacolin K—a compound chemically identical to lovastatin[36], the first statin drug used to lower cholesterol. In China and other Asian countries, it is traditionally used as a medicine. The main ingredient is monacolin K. The commercial varieties of red yeast rice have varying quantities of this active compound. It has been used in the management of high cholesterol disorders if patients do not tolerate drug therapy. The US Food and Drug Administration (FDA) has advised against the use of this supplement. Recently, kidney injury due to red yeast rice has been reported from Japan.[37] If used at all, a physician's supervision is required.

How to Parboil Paddy (Unhusked Rice)? A Process Prior to De-Husking

Parboiled rice (*sela chawal*) is usually produced on an industrial scale, where rice kernels are subjected to a parboiling process before de-husking. Method (traditional/home-scale):

1. In a saucepan, boil water and add salt and olive oil (optional) to it.
2. When the water comes to a rolling boil, add the paddy (unhusked rice) and let it come to a boil again.
3. Cook the paddy on medium-high heat for 5–10 minutes.
4. Now drain the paddy. Return the paddy to the pan and cover.
5. Rinse with cold water and let it dry.
6. Remove the husk with hands or in the mill.
7. Store in a cool and dry place.

Summary Statement Regarding *Roti*s and Rice

This statement is for all people and specifically for those with diabetes. In India, *roti*s and rice are staple foods. To make wheat flour healthier and more nutritious, it should be mixed with other flours (*besan,* pearl millet [*bajra*] or barley [*jau*]) to make *chapati*s. These mixed-flour *chapati*s provide additional fibre, protein and micronutrients, making them a healthier alternative to plain wheat *chapati*s. Similarly, rice like brown rice (*bhura chawal*) and parboiled rice (*sela chawal*) are healthier varieties and may be better for people with diabetes as compared to white rice.

TABLE 5.4 Comparison of Nutritive Values of Different Types of Cooked Rice (All values are per 100 g portion)

		White Rice (*safed chawal*)	Brown Rice (*bhura chawal*)	Parboiled White Rice (*sela chawal*)	Glutinous White Rice (*chipchipa chawal*)	Sprouted Brown Rice (*ankurit bhura chawal*)
Energy	Cal	143	162	123	97	220
Macronutrients						
Protein	g	2.86	3.81	2.91	2.02	4
Fat	g	0	1.43	0.37	0.19	2
Carbohydrate	g	31.4	34.29	26.05	21.09	50
Fibre	g	0	1.9	0.9	1	2
Micronutrients						
Thiamine	mg			0.212 (10% of RDA)	0.02	0
Niacin	mg			2.3 (23% of RDA)	0.29	3.2
Vitamin B_6	mg			0.15 (14% of RDA)	0.026	-
GI		73	68	46	48	55

Source: Author's own compilation.
Any differences in nutrient values reflect variations in data sources, analytical methods and preparation methods.

Vegetables

Bitter Gourd (Momordica charantia, karela)

Bitter gourd is a vegetable that is popularly eaten as a part of vegetarian meals in India. It is green and oblong.

Nutrition Facts

A serving of 100 g contains 4.32 g carbs (2 g fibre), 0.18 g fat and 0.84 g protein (these values may vary depending on the source). It contains a high concentration of vitamin C and 7 percent potassium, among multiple other vitamins and minerals.

Popular Health-Centric Uses

Traditionally, bitter gourd (*karela*) has been used to treat abdominal and respiratory diseases and is popular in the treatment of type 2 diabetes. It is also sold as herbal tea.

Scientific Studies

1. Mostly, bitter gourd has been used as an adjunctive treatment to main diabetes therapy. Most studies that show its glucose-lowering properties are small and scientifically inadequate. It is stated to increase insulin secretion and glucose utilisation in peripheral tissues, but more research is required.[38]
2. Some studies have shown its potential as an anti-obesity drug.[39]
3. Its effects on inflammation and cancer have been explored but need additional research.

Fenugreek

Fenugreek (*Trigonella foenum-graecum*; *methi*) is a part of traditional Indian culinary practices. Fenugreek has leaves consisting of three small obovate to oblong leaflets, and its seeds and leaves are common ingredients in dishes from South and Central Asia.

Nutrition Facts

One serving of 100 g fenugreek seeds (*methi*) contains 323 Cal, 58 g carbs (25 g fibre) 6.4 g fat, 23 g protein and multiple vitamins and minerals (these values may vary depending on the source). Phytochemical analysis reveals the presence of steroids, alkaloids, saponins, polyphenols, flavonoids, lipids, carbohydrates, amino acids and hydrocarbons.

Popular Health-Centric Uses

Ingestion of fenugreek is perceived to be healthy. Many believe in the antidiabetic property of fenugreek.

Scientific Studies

1. Despite its popularity as a 'healthy' dietary ingredient, scientific studies are limited. In a few studies, it has been shown to decrease blood glucose levels. Its lipid-lowering property, though demonstrated in some studies, remains to be proven.[40] Based on current information, it can be used only as an adjuvant to the main therapy of type 2 diabetes while monitoring blood sugar levels carefully.
2. It has been used in neurological disorders and depression, but more research is needed.[41]

How Can Fenugreek Be Used?

Soaked fenugreek seeds can be taken with hot water. The prescribed dose of fenugreek varies from 25 to 50 g (2–3 tbsp). Ideally, to begin with, 25 g of the seeds may be given in two doses of 12.5 g each (about 1 tbsp) along with meals. They can be worked into *chapatis*, rice, lentils (*dal*), vegetables, curd (*dahi*), pickle *(achaar)*, *chutneys* or sprouts in salad.

Safety

Rarely, it may cause allergies. It has the potential to cause abdominal upset. It may increase the potency of blood thinner drugs.

Jackfruit

Jackfruit (*kathal*) is a fruit commonly eaten in India and Malaysia.

Nutrition Facts

One serving of 100 g of edible ripe jackfruit flesh (95 Cal) has 24 g carbs (1.6 g fibre), 0.3 g fats and 1.47 g protein. It also contains vitamin B_6, vitamin A, vitamin C and potassium (these values may vary depending on the source).

Scientific Studies

1. Animal studies showed that extracts of jackfruit improved glucose tolerance in normal individuals and patients with diabetes.[42] A randomised trial showed that jackfruit flour significantly decreases blood glucose values in patients with type 2 diabetes as compared to the placebo.[43] Since it was a twelve-week trial in a limited number of patients, more trials are needed.
2. There are some preliminary studies that show that jackfruit may have anti-inflammatory and antioxidant properties.[44]

Mushrooms (kukurmutta)

Mushrooms grow on surfaces or feed on another source. There are numerous varieties, some of which are edible. Mushrooms are used in European, Chinese, Japanese and, increasingly, Indian cooking.

Nutrition Facts

One serving of brown mushrooms (100 g) contains 22 Cal energy, 4.3 g carbohydrate, 0.1 g fat, 2.5 g protein and a good amount of B vitamins, potassium, selenium and zinc (these values may vary depending on the source).

Popular Health-Centric Uses

Certain mushroom species, particularly those containing psilocybin and related compounds, exhibit psychoactive properties and have historically been used in spiritual or ritual contexts for perceived healing. These mushrooms can induce psychedelic experiences, including altered perception, mood and cognition. In modern psychiatry, psilocybin is being studied as a potential treatment for conditions such as treatment-resistant depression, anxiety, post-traumatic stress disorder (PTSD) and substance use disorders, though clinical use remains experimental and tightly regulated. Mushrooms have also been used in Chinese medicines.

Scientific Studies

1. Although studies are not conclusive, anti-tumour, anti-inflammatory, anti-oxidative and antibacterial properties have been shown.[45]

2. There is some evidence from China that the intake of mushrooms can significantly lower the risk of cognitive decline in older adults.[46]
3. They have low GI, and hence, it is useful to include them in food planning of patients with diabetes (especially oyster mushrooms).[47]
4. However, the number of modern chemical, biological and pharmacological studies remains limited, and several mushroom species remain entirely unstudied. Moreover, there is a lack of valid clinical studies to support their therapeutic use.

Caution

1. Several mushrooms are poisonous, and it may be difficult to segregate them from edible mushrooms. Those mushrooms may cause allergy, asthma-like symptoms and even allergic shock (anaphylactic shock). So it is better to purchase them from a reliable source.
2. Cultivated mushrooms *also* contain small amounts of hydrazine, which is a toxin. However, it is destroyed by heat.

Asparagus (Asparagus officinalis)

Asparagus is a flowering plant. Its young shoots are used as a spring vegetable. *Asparagus racemosus* (*satavar, shatavari, shatamull* or *shatawari*) is a species of asparagus common throughout Nepal, Sri Lanka, India and the Himalayas.

Nutrition Facts

A 100 g serving of asparagus provides about 20 Cal, 3.9 g carbohydrates (including 2.1 g fibre and 1.9 g sugars), 2.2 g protein and 0.1 g fat. It is rich in potassium with small amounts of sodium and an excellent source of folate, vitamin K, thiamine and riboflavin (these values may vary depending on the source).

Popular Health-Centric Uses

Asparagus is eaten as a vegetable owing to its distinct flavour and used in medicine due to its diuretic properties. *Asparagus racemosus* is recommended in Ayurvedic texts for prevention and treatment of gastric ulcers (curative effect in patients of duodenal ulcers) and dyspepsia (promotes gastric emptying). It is also a galactagogue (helps in increasing milk secretion during lactation). It has also been used successfully for nervous disorders, inflammation, liver diseases and certain infectious diseases to consolidate these findings.

Scientific Studies

1. Evidence in animal studies suggests that *Asparagus adscendens* (*shweta musali*) has insulin-enhancing activity.[48] These actions are dependent on the active principle(s) in the plant being absorbed intact. More studies are needed to consolidate these findings.
2. Future work assessing its use as a dietary adjunct or as a source of active components may provide new opportunities for the treatment of diabetes. *Asparagus racemosus* may be useful as a source of novel antidiabetic compounds or a dietary adjunct for the management of diabetes.[49]
3. The extract of asparagus stem, when treated with enzyme, could alleviate stress, promote quality of sleep and decrease fatigue in otherwise healthy individuals.[50]

How Can Asparagus Be Used?

It is eaten as a vegetable. The seed and root extracts of asparagus are used in alcoholic beverages. In Asian-style cooking, asparagus is often fried. It may also be used as an ingredient in some stews and soups. In recent years, asparagus, eaten raw as a component of a salad, has regained popularity.

Okra (Abelmoschus esculentus, ladies' fingers, bhindi, vendakkai)

Okra (*bhindi*) is a long, tapering edible seed pod, commonly available in South Asia and other parts of the world.

Nutrition Facts

One serving of 100 g raw okra contains about 35 Cal, 7 g carbohydrates (3 g fibre), 0.2 g fat, 1.9 g protein. It is high in vitamins C and K and provides good amounts of folate, thiamine and magnesium (these values may vary depending on the source).

Popular Health-Centric Uses

Okra is perceived to be a healthy food and good for weight loss. Okra water, peels and powdered seeds are used for health purposes.

Scientific Studies

1. Scientific studies are preliminary and suggest blood glucose–lowering properties, similar to drugs of the class 'alpha-glucosidase inhibitor' (tablets such as acarbose are used for treatment of type 2 diabetes).[51]
2. Animal studies also show benefit in gestational diabetes.[52] There are no human studies.
3. As the okra pod contains a good amount of protein, fibre, calcium, iron and zinc, increase in its consumption may help alleviate malnutrition-related deficiencies.[53]

Lotus Stem and Root (Nelumbo nucifera, kamal kakdi, bhein, nadru)

Lotus stem (*kamal kakdi*) is the edible (underground stem) of the lotus plant. It is consumed in India, China, Japan and Southeast Asia, especially in Kashmiri cuisine. It has a mildly sweet, crunchy texture and is used in a variety of preparations such as curries, pickles *(achaar)* and stir fries.

Nutrition Facts

One 100 g serving of lotus stem provides about 74 Cal energy, 17 g carbohydrates, 4.9 g of fibre, 0.1 g of fat and 2.6 g protein. It is a good source of dietary fibre, vitamin C, potassium and manganese and contains modest amounts of B_6, copper and phosphorus (these values may vary depending on the source).

Popular Health-Centric Uses

Lotus stem is considered a digestive aid in traditional Indian and Chinese systems of medicine. It is thought to support gut health and immunity. It is also consumed for its potential to manage diarrhoea, improve circulation and act as a cooling agent during fever. Lotus stem flour is sometimes used in diabetic diets due to its fibre and resistant starch content.

Scientific Studies

1. Blood glucose effects: A few *in vitro* and animal studies suggest lotus root may help lower postprandial blood glucose via inhibition of digestive enzymes (for example, α amylase), though human data is lacking.[54]

2. Antioxidant and anti-inflammatory properties: Lotus rhizome is rich in polyphenols, including catechins and caffeine acid derivatives, with demonstrated antioxidant and anti-inflammatory activity *in vitro*.[55] These may have long-term benefits in chronic diseases.
3. Anti-obesity and lipid effects: Animal studies show lotus root extracts may reduce adipose tissue inflammation and improve lipid profile in high-fat diet–fed rodents.[56] Evidence in humans is not available.
4. Other benefits: Traditional use as an astringent and haemostatic agent in Ayurvedic and Unani systems is well established, but scientific validation is minimal.

Potatoes (Solanum tuberosum, aaloo)

Potato is a tuber of the plant. There are 500 natural varieties of potatoes (*aaloo*) as well as genetically engineered varieties.

Nutrition Facts

One serving of 100 g potatoes contains 84 Cal energy, 17 g carbohydrates (2.2 g fibre, 0.78 g sugar), 0.1 g fat, 2 g protein, high vitamin C, and it is a good source of potassium (these values may vary depending on the source). About 50 percent of the fibre is located in or just under the skin.

Popular Health-Centric Uses

Potatoes generally have negative health implications. It is popularly believed that eating potatoes increases blood sugar levels and increases weight. Hence, the intake of potatoes is believed to be bad for health.

Scientific Studies

In general, moderate consumption of potatoes, when included as part of a balanced diet, is acceptable for people with or without diabetes and hypertension. However, large intakes, particularly of fried potatoes or potato chips, can be detrimental due to their high glycaemic impact, added fats and potential for harmful compounds such as acrylamide. Key studies evaluating the effects of potato consumption on blood glucose, body weight and cardiovascular health are summarised below:

1. A major analysis concludes that eating potatoes is not related to an increased risk of death.[57 58]
2. Total potato consumption has not been linked to deaths due to heart attack.[59]
3. There is a greater feeling of satiety (stomach fullness) on eating potatoes.[60]
4. There is no conclusive data to link potatoes to high risk of diabetes, although risk is more with French fries (*tale hue aaloo*).[61] Although this association has been contested[62], recent research substantiates these findings. Three servings of French fries per week raised type 2 diabetes risk by almost 20 percent, whereas whole grain substitution reduced the risk by up to 19 percent. Meta-analysis confirmed elevated type 2 diabetes risk mainly for fried potato (*tale hue aaloo*) products, not non-fried forms.[63]
5. Potatoes have a high GI value (70–90) that can increase blood sugar response, but some varieties may also have low values. The GI values of potatoes vary according to the variety and cooking method used:[64 65]
   i. Boiled red potatoes (*uble hue laal aaloo*) consumed cold: intermediate
   ii. Roasted California white potatoes (*safed aaloo*) and baked US Russet potatoes: moderately high
   iii. Instant mashed potatoes and boiled red potatoes: high
6. Higher intake of baked, boiled or mashed potatoes and French fries was independently and prospectively associated with an increased risk of developing hypertension.[66]

Fried Potatoes and French Fries

1. Potatoes can be consumed fried, and a popular variant of fried potatoes is French fries.
2. Consumption of fried potatoes has been linked to early death and diabetes.[58]
3. French fries, when cooked in partially hydrogenated vegetable oils (for example, *vanaspati ghee*), which is full of trans-fatty acids, are bad for the heart and blood vessels. The levels of trans-fats in French fries varies depending on the oil used.

4. French fries also contains acrylamide, which is a probable human carcinogen that is not naturally present but develops while frying. The darker and crispier the fries, the higher the acrylamide content.[67]

Fried Potato Chips

1. Fried potato chips also contain acrylamide. The presence of acrylamide has been shown in several commercial chips sold in South India.[68]
2. Ingestion of potato chips for even four weeks increases bad oxidised radicals and inflammation, likely due to acrylamide.[69]

Caution

Damaged potatoes, green potatoes (*hara aaloo*) and sprouts may have some poisonous chemicals that can cause nausea, vomiting, diarrhoea and abdominal pain.

Sweet Potato (Ipomoea batatas, shakarakand)

Sweet potato (*shakarakand*) is a sweet-tasting root vegetable.

Nutrition Facts

One serving of 100 g cooked sweet potato provides approximately 90 Cal, 20 g carbohydrates (about 6 g sugars, 3 g fibre, 7 g starch), 0.1 g fat and approximately 2 g protein. It is very high in vitamin A (as beta-carotene) and also provides vitamin B_6, vitamin C, manganese, potassium and vitamin K (these values may vary depending on the source).

Popular Health-Centric Uses

Sweet potatoes are believed to be good for eye health and digestion. Because of the sweet taste and high content of carbs, these are perceived to be bad for patients with diabetes.

Scientific Studies

1. The nutritional value of sweet potatoes is among the highest among several foods, particularly because of the high content of beta-carotene and vitamin A. Indeed, its widespread use

has been recommended in sub-Saharan Africa for vitamin A deficiency.[70]

2. Tuber and leaves have been used for experimental studies for diabetes. In a Cochrane review (a highly respected scientific source), all controlled trials of sweet potatoes in diabetes were considered for analysis. Some trials showed improved blood sugar control with the ingestion of sweet potatoes. The authors of the Cochrane review stated: 'There is insufficient evidence to recommend use of sweet potato for type 2 diabetes.'[71]
3. Some data shows its effects on weight loss (as meal replacement) and on blood arteries.[72]

How Can Sweet Potato Be Used?

Sweet potatoes can be eaten as a boiled or pressure-cooked snack or with the main meal. When dried, it can be ground to make bread (*chapatis*). It is also used to make pickles (*achaar*), snacks and chips.

Tomatoes (Solanum lycopersicum, tamatar)

Tomato (*tamatar*) is a red berry from the tomato plant.

Nutrition Facts

One serving of 100 g raw tomatoes contains 18 Cal energy, 3.9 g carbohydrates (2.6 g sugars, 1.2 g fibre) 0.2 g fat and 0.9 g protein. It is a good source of vitamin C and contains a high amount of lycopene.

What Is Lycopene?

A bright-red carotenoid hydrocarbon, lycopene is found in large amounts in tomatoes, red carrots (*gajar*), watermelons (*tarbooz*), pink grapefruits (*chakotara*) and papayas (*papita*). Tomato ketchup has a good amount of lycopene.

Scientific Studies

Lycopene and α-tomatine are reported to have health-promoting effects, including anti-cancer and heart protection activities. Most published reports have attributed effects, if any, to lycopene.[73] None have been conclusively proven.

1. Tomato intake has been shown to decrease body inflammatory markers.[74] [75]

2. Some data shows that body damage/photo damage induced by solar radiation could be prevented by tomatoes/lycopene.[76]
3. Tomato intake has been shown to be associated with less prostate cancer in some studies. This was not substantiated in a major review.[77]
4. Some positive effects on blood lipids and blood pressure have been shown.[78]
5. Good effects of tomatoes on several brain disorders, including memory and cognition, have been hypothesised.[79]
6. A study shows that tomato and lycopene consumption is inversely associated with death rates and heart attacks.[80]

Caution

Lycopene (commercial) or a high number of tomatoes should not be consumed before surgery as it may increase the risk of bleeding.

Carrot (Daucus carota subsp. sativus, gajar)

Carrot is a root vegetable.

Nutrition Facts

One 100 g serving of raw carrots (*gajar*) provides 41 Cal, 9.6 g carbohydrates (including 4.7 g sugars and 2.8 g fibre), 0.9 g protein and just 0.2 g fat. Carrots are an excellent source of vitamin A and beta-carotene, which gives them their bright orange colour (these values may vary depending on the source). Beta-carotene is a precursor (inactive form) to vitamin A.

Popular Health-Centric Uses

Carrots are perceived as healthy and good for eyesight.

What Is Beta-carotene and Where Is It Found?

Beta-carotene is a pigment found in palm oil (contains highest amount of beta-carotene), mangoes (*aam*), pumpkin (*kaddu*), papaya (*papita*) and sweet potatoes (*shakarakand*). It is converted to vitamin A in the body.

Scientific Studies

The following are the effects of beta-carotene:

1. It has good antioxidant activity.

2. High blood levels of beta-carotene biochemical status are associated with overall lower incidence of cardiovascular disease, heart disease, stroke, cancer and other causes of mortality according to a recent major analysis.[81]
3. Some concern has been raised that intake of beta-carotene increases the risk of lung cancer in cigarette smokers and these people should avoid eating carrots. Increase in lung cancer is only found when high doses of beta-carotene were used.[82] It may increase lung cancer risk when used for prevention.[83]
4. Similarly, for those with exposure to asbestos, it may increase lung cancer risk. High doses are also likely to increase risk of death.[84]
5. There may be some protective effects of beta-carotene on cataracts.[85]
6. There is conflicting evidence of its use in age-related macular degeneration.
7. It is used for treatment of an inherited disorder of skin sensitivity to light (porphyria).[86]

Carotenemia

High amounts of carrot intake can cause yellow discoloration of the skin.

Maize (bhutta/makka)

Maize refers to the cereal corn kernels attached to a grass stalk. It can be consumed in various ways, including eating the kernels directly or in processed forms such as popcorn, sweetcorn and more.

Nutrition Facts

One serving of 100 g maize (*bhutta*) contains 96 Cal energy, 20 g carbohydrates (4.5 g sugars, 2.7 g fibre), 1.2 g fat and 3.2 g protein (these values may vary depending on the source). It also contains pantothenic acid, niacin, folate, manganese, phosphorus, lutein and zeaxanthin. One *bhutta* has 100 Cal.

Popular Health-Centric Uses

Maize is considered beneficial for eye health and digestion. However, due to its sweet taste and high carbohydrate content, it is often perceived by most people as unsuitable for patients with diabetes.[87]

Scientific Studies

Most studies are concerned with the metabolic effects of corn oil (discussed separately) or high-fructose corn syrup (see section on 'Sugar, Sugar-Related Beverages and Artificial Sweeteners'). Very few studies are available regarding the effect of corn kernels or their preparation on blood glucose levels in humans. In one study, the glucose response elicited from the consumption of wheat, rice and corn muffins was comparable but significantly greater when compared with oat (*jai*) and barley (*jau*) muffins.[88]

How Is Corn Used?

Corn is consumed as food, snacks, corn syrup, popcorn (see page 164), cornflakes, sweetcorn and so on. Corn is also used to make bourbon and as animal fodder.

Broccoli

Broccoli (*brokolee*) is a green plant belonging to the cabbage (*patta gobhi*) family.

Nutrition Facts

One serving of 100 g raw broccoli contains 34 Cal, 6.64 g carbs (1.7 g sugar, 2.6 g fibre), 0.35 g fats and 2.82 g protein. It is rich in vitamin C and vitamin K with good amounts of folate, potassium and iron (these values may vary depending on the source).

Popular Health-Centric Uses

In India, broccoli is not widely consumed but is perceived as a healthy dietary choice.

Scientific Studies

Broccoli has a strong scientific background to be classified as a health-promoting nutrient. Broccoli is rich in vitamins, minerals and isothiocyanates, sulforaphane being the most important nutrient.

1. It has been shown to lower blood cholesterol levels.[89]
2. Sulforaphane has been shown to possess anti-inflammatory and anti-cancer properties.[90]

3. Intake of broccoli offers protection against environmental pollution. Specifically, it causes detoxication of benzene, an important airborne pollutant.[91]
4. In a randomised trial, broccoli extract has been shown to improve liver functions in humans with fatty liver and animals with liver failure.[92]
5. A trial shows that broccoli sprout extract may lower blood sugar levels.[93]

Spinach (Spinacia oleracea)

The leaves of the spinach plant (*paalak*) are eaten cooked or raw.

Nutrition Facts

1. Per 100 g, spinach provides 23 Cal, 3.6 g carbohydrates (0.4 g sugars, 2.2 g fibre), 2.9 g protein and 0.4 g fat. It is especially rich in vitamin K and beta-carotene and also supplies folate, vitamin C, magnesium, manganese and iron (these values may vary depending on the source).
2. Raw spinach contains a high amount of oxalate, which may block iron absorption. Several washings of spinach may decrease oxalate content.
3. Spinach has a high content of nitrates.

Popular Health-Centric Uses

The legend of the health benefits of spinach has been propagated by the famous cartoon character Popeye, who gains strength upon eating spinach. While this depiction is well-meaning, the claim is somewhat exaggerated, as the actual nutritional impact, though beneficial, does not confer instantaneous superhuman strength.

Scientific Studies

1. As it is a low-calorie yet filling food, it is ideal for patients with diabetes and obesity.
2. The nitrate content of spinach eases the blood flow of the arteries.[94] This may benefit the cardiovascular system.
3. Consumption of spinach stabilises damage to DNA due to any cause. This may have implications for chronic diseases and cancers.[95]

4. A systematic review of four RCTs (ninety-four participants) found improvements in most performance measures, with mixed effects on body composition. Further research is needed to define optimal dosing and effects across different populations.[96]

Caution

1. Patients who are on the anticoagulant warfarin should avoid eating spinach because of its high vitamin K content, which negates the effect of warfarin.
2. It may cause crystal deposition in the kidneys.

Beans

Beans (*phaliyan*) are seeds from several flowering plants. There are several beans available in India, and their classification may cause some confusion. The following is a representative list:

1. Black-eyed bean (*chawli, lobia*)
2. Kidney beans (*rajma*): popular and commonly cooked in North India
3. Adjuki beans (*chori*)
4. Dew gram beans (*matki*)
5. Lentils (*masoor, arhar, chana, urad* and so on): broken seeds of lentils

Nutrition Facts

1. Beans, in general, are rich in protein, complex carbs, fibre (one cup has 13 g), vitamins (folate) and iron. Per 100 g, kidney beans (*rajma*) contain about 333 Cal, 60 g carbohydrates (including approximately 2 g sugars and 15 g fibre), 24 g protein and 1 g fat. It is a rich source of folate, magnesium, potassium, iron, phosphorus and manganese.
2. They have low GI and are, hence, suitable for people with diabetes.

Scientific Studies

1. Polyphenols in beans have antioxidant properties. Common beans (*Phaseolus vulgaris L.*; the red type is *rajma*) are a greater source of polyphenolic compounds with numerous health-promoting properties. Polyphenol-rich dry common beans have potential effects on human health and possess

antioxidant, anti-diabetic, anti-obesity, anti-inflammatory, anti-mutagenic and anti-carcinogenic properties.[97]

2. Black beans (*kale rajma*) or chickpeas (*kabuli chana/desi chana*) consumed with white rice significantly lowered post-meal blood glucose compared to rice alone in healthy women. These findings support incorporating legumes into traditional meals to improve glycaemic control and reduce related health risks.[98]
3. Iron fortification of beans has been tried to increase iron status in people with anaemia.[99]
4. There is some evidence that intake of canned beans (*phali*) may lower cholesterol levels.[100]
5. In one study, several legumes were studied—cowpeas, mung beans, pole sitao, chickpeas (*chole*), green peas, groundnuts, pigeon peas, kidney beans (*rajma*), lima beans and soybeans. They showed variable mineral availability and were all low-GI foods. Some (kidney beans, groundnuts [*moongphali*]) reduced cholesterol, supporting their role as functional foods for chronic disease prevention.[101]

Garlic (Allium sativum)

Garlic (*lahsun*) is a tuber of a plant and is frequently eaten mixed with various foods.

Nutrition Facts

Per 100 g, garlic contains 149 Cal, 33 g carbohydrates (1 g sugar, 2.1 g fibre), 6.4 g protein and 0.5 g fat and is rich in vitamin B_6, vitamin C and manganese (these values may vary depending on the source).

Popular Health-Centric Uses

1. Garlic is perceived as a healthy and heart-friendly food and is taken raw daily by many people in India. Although it is widely believed to have several 'heart-friendly' properties, many of these claims remain scientifically unproven.
2. It has been used as an antibacterial agent (frequently used in the First World War).

Scientific Studies

1. Garlic has been used for prevention and management of hypertension and heart disease. It has been shown to reduce

blood pressure in a small measure.[102] Overall data regarding these uses is not convincing.

2. It has been shown to decrease inflammation.[103]
3. The effect of garlic on cholesterol levels has been much advertised, and many commercial preparations are made with garlic. Although data is conflicting, a recent meta-analysis shows that garlic lowers lipids as well as blood glucose in people with diabetes to some extent.[104] However, one should never replace cholesterol-lowering drugs (statins, which have many heart-friendly actions, other than cholesterol-lowering) with commercial garlic preparations.
4. It may have some anti-cancer effects, particularly against cancer of the upper intestine.[105]
5. It may have some anti-inflammatory properties and has been shown to reduce pain in knee arthritis.[106]
6. It has some effects on coagulation-forming blood cells (platelets).[107] [108]

Fruits and Berries

Since a variety of fruits are available, none of them are described in detail here. A common question often asked by patients with diabetes is which fruit and how much can be eaten. It is generally fine to eat one fruit daily. One could choose among those listed in Table 5.5.

TABLE 5.5 Glycaemic Index and Glycaemic Load of Various Fruits

Fruits	Weight (g)	Calories (Cal)	GI	GI Ranking	GL	GL Ranking
Strawberries (*stroberee*)	100 (1 cup)	33	40	Low	1	Low
Cherries (*cheree*)	72 (1 cup)	46	22	Low	3	Low
Pear (*nashpati*)	100 (1 whole)	52	38	Low	4	Low
Peach (*aadu*)	100 (1 whole)	50	42	Low	5	Low
Orange (*santra*)	100 (1 medium)	44	44	Low	5	Low
Apricots (*khubani*)	100	48	31	Low	5	Low
Apple (*seb*)	75 (1 whole)	44	38	Low	6	Low

Fruits	Weight (g)	Calories (Cal)	GI	GI Ranking	GL	GL Ranking
Plum (*aaloo bukhara*)	30 (1 whole)	31	39	Low	7	Low
Musk melon (*kharbooja*)	100 (1 cup)	34	65	Intermediate	4	Low
Mango (*aam*)	60 (1 medium)	44	56	Intermediate	5	Low
Kiwifruit (*kiwi*)	69 (1 whole)	42	58	Intermediate	5	Low
Pineapple (*anaanaas*)	100 (1 cup)	46	66	Intermediate	7	Low
Papaya (*papita*)	100 (1 cup)	44	58	Intermediate	10	Low
Wood apple (*bael*)	100	110	57	Intermediate	10	Low
Guava (*amrood*)	100 (1 whole)	68	78	High	4	Low
Watermelon (*tarbooz*)	100 (1 cup)	49	72	High	4	Low
Grapes (*angoor*)	100 (1 cup)	43	59	Intermediate	11	Intermediate
Banana (*kela*)	1 medium	95	55	Intermediate	16	Intermediate
Figs, dried (*anjeer*)	1 piece	30	61	Intermediate	25	High

Source: Author's own compilation.
Any differences in nutrient values reflect variations in data sources, analytical methods and preparation methods.

Easy Reading 9
Should I Eat Mangoes?

1. Mango is considered the 'king of Asian fruits' and is the national fruit of India. Eating mangoes is generally considered to be bad for patients with diabetes and obesity. Both patients and physicians often blame intake of mangoes for weight gain and high blood sugar levels.
2. GI of mangoes: There is confusion regarding its nutritional and glycaemic values. Mangoes are often considered as

having high GI and GL. Glycaemic values of mango are not high at all! Its (120 g mango) GI is 51 and GL is 8, both of which are categorised as low.

3. In the past few years, there has been increasing interest in the study of mango fruits, peels, seeds and stem bark due to their anti-oxidative and health-promoting properties. Some studies show that mango consumption reduced overall blood glucose levels. However, these studies have been done in a small number of patients and mostly in other countries.
4. So is mango totally safe as a fruit? Can we take it regularly? These questions have not been answered yet. Across two studies carried out by us, replacing bread with mango for breakfast led to similar or lower post-meal glucose levels as compared to bread, reduced glycaemic variability (glucose level variations) and improved metabolism in people with type 2 diabetes. Benefits included lower fasting glucose, glycosylated haemoglobin (indicates average blood glucose), insulin resistance, body weight, waist circumference and higher HDL cholesterol.[109 110]
5. My statement, based on our research, is 'we showed the benefits of small doses of mangoes in place of carbohydrates (bread) in breakfast in two detailed studies for the first time, laying to rest all speculations regarding adverse metabolic effects of its consumption ... However, these must be incorporated into diets of people with diabetes under strict supervision of nutritionists—within prescribed limits and not in excess—and aligned to the individual's clinical profile, as judged by physicians.'

Jamun (Syzygium cumini/jambul/black plum/java plum/Indian blackberry)

Jamun is a purple-black fruit (berry) commonly available in summers in India (Figure 5.2).

Nutrition Facts

One serving of 100 g of raw *jamun* contains approximately 60 Cal, 15 g carbohydrates (0.6 g fibre), 0.2 g fat, 0.7–1 g protein and around 84 g water (these values may vary depending on the source).

Popular Health-Centric Uses

Jamun is commonly perceived as good for people with diabetes and believed to aid in digestion.

Scientific Studies

1. There are several studies in experimental animals that show the glucose-lowering effect of *jamun*.[111]
2. Unfortunately, only a few studies are available in humans. In a small, randomised trial with *S. cumini* tea in patients with diabetes in Brazil, no effect on blood glucose levels was observed.[112]
3. It can inhibit toxic advanced glycosylation end products (harmful products) in people with diabetes.[113]
4. It also has alpha-glucosidase inhibitor activity (similar activity to a drug, acarbose, used in the treatment of diabetes), but more research is needed.
5. However, one study also shows that its seeds could be toxic to the liver in experimental animals.[114]

How Can *Jamun* Be Used?

Jamun is eaten as a berry or powder. It is used to make juices and jams and is mixed in ice cream or smoothies. It could be taken as a dietary adjunct in patients with diabetes.

Other Berries

These are small, juicy fruits (Figure 5.2). These are eaten fresh and also as a part of jams, cakes, pastries and the like.

Nutrition Facts

Berries (skins, leaves and seeds) contain anthocyanins and flavonoids and have antioxidant properties. Berries also contain good amounts of fibre, vitamins and minerals. There are very few scientific studies to support health benefits.

1. Strawberries have been shown to alleviate pain in knee arthritis (osteoarthritis, knee joint affected due to age).[115]

2. Resveratrol (mainly found in grapes [*angoor*], red wine, peanuts [*moongphali*], cranberries [*karonda*], pistachios [*pista*], blueberries [*neelbadri*] and bilberries [*jangli blueberry*]) may have benefits for the cardiovascular system and inflammation.[116] Blueberries are rich in anthocyanins (see next section). They show anti-inflammatory and antioxidant actions and may benefit heart and glucose metabolism. Blueberries may also affect gut flora.
3. Intake of berries may positively affect bones.[117]

Blueberries (blooberee/neelbadri/neela jamun)

Blueberries (genus *Vaccinium*) are edible blue-purple berries. These are not usually sold by fruit vendors in India. They are used as fresh and dried fruits in juices and jams.

Nutrition Facts

One serving of 100 g blueberries provides about 57 Cal, 9.9 g sugars and 2.4 g fibre. It is high in vitamin C and other micronutrients, and contains approximately 84 g water. Blueberries contain anthocyanins (water-soluble pigments) and phytochemicals (these values may vary depending on the source).

Popular Health-Centric Uses

Blueberries are perceived as healthy fruits, but consumption in India is low because of non-availability and prohibitive cost.

Scientific Studies

1. Blueberries have been termed as one of the best functional foods. The potential health benefits (antioxidant, anti-inflammatory) of blueberries may be due to the effects of anthocyanins on blood vessels.[118]
2. Berries such as blueberries, bilberries (*jangli blueberry*) and cranberries (*karonda*) are natural sources of resveratrol (as mentioned earlier), a compound with antioxidant, anti-inflammatory and blood glucose-lowering properties and multiple beneficial effects on other organs.[116]
3. Even short-term ingestion of blueberries has been shown to decrease blood pressure. This may be due to an increase in nitrous oxide production.[119]

4. Through the effects on small vessels (endothelium) and inflammation, they have the potential to improve cardiovascular health.[118 120]
5. Other effects include improvement in blood glucose and cholesterol levels.[121]
6. Some studies have shown improvement in memory with the consumption of blueberries.[122] However, more robust studies are required.
7. Consumption of blueberries increased the number of muscle cells in women, thus showing potential to improve muscle functions.[123]

Use of Blueberries

Blueberries can be eaten as snacks or as part of fruit cocktails. Per day, 25–100 g can be taken.

Indian Gooseberry (amla/Emblica officinalis/Phyllanthus emblica)

Indian gooseberry (*amla*) is a fruit. This tree is cultivated commonly in India, Sri Lanka, China and Malaysia.

Nutrition Facts

One serving of 100 g *amla* (15 pieces) contains 48 Cal energy, 14 g carbohydrates (1.9 g fibre), 0.1 g fat and 0.5 g protein and is exceptionally rich in vitamin C, along with some vitamin A (these values may vary depending on the source).

Popular Health-Centric Uses

Indian gooseberry has been effectively used in many Ayurveda formulations, specially to enhance digestion as well as to treat constipation. It is known to be rich in vitamin C.

Scientific Studies

1. The *amla* fruit has thirty times more vitamin C than an orange. Most of the studies done using amla are small and not robust. The bioactivities of *amla* are ascribed to polyphenols (tannins, flavonoids), which can have antioxidant and immunomodulator properties.

2. One randomised trial shows that extract of *amla* (500 mg twice daily) when given for twelve weeks can lower triglycerides and cholesterol (blood fats).[124]
3. In a study on rats, *amla* extract (contains ellagic acid, also present in various fruits and nuts—particularly pomegranates, strawberries, raspberries, blackberries and walnuts) was shown to increase insulin secretion by activating beta cells of the pancreas.[125 126]
4. A meta-analysis shows that use of *amla* reduces inflammation, blood sugar and lipids.[127]
5. In a research study, both atorvastatin (a powerful lipid-lowering drug that can protect against heart attacks) and aqueous extract of *amla* significantly improved endothelial (inner lining of arteries) function and reduced biomarkers of oxidative stress and systemic inflammation in people with type 2 diabetes.[128]
6. *Amla* may have additional benefits, including beneficial effects on nerve damage due to diabetes (diabetic neuropathy).[129] Gooseberry also has a blood-thinning action (anti-platelet action), but this needs confirmation. Some beneficial effect on cataracts has also been seen but needs confirmation in human studies.[130]

How Can *Amla* Be Used?

Amla can be consumed fresh or dried and is used to prepare candies, fruit preserve (*murabba*), sherbet, juice, digestive powder (*churan*), pickles (*achaar*) and *chutneys*.

FIGURE 5.2 Various Types of Berries Available in India

Images of Various Berries	English/Hindi Name
1. 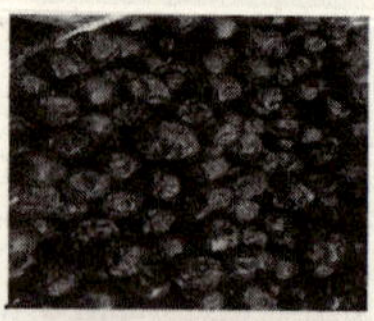	Cranberry (*karonda/phalse*): 1 *katori* (100 g) = 46 Cal
2. 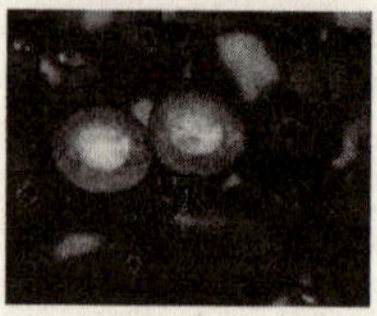	Indian blackberry (*jamun*): 1 *katori* (100 g) = 62 Cal

Images of Various Berries	English/Hindi Name
3. 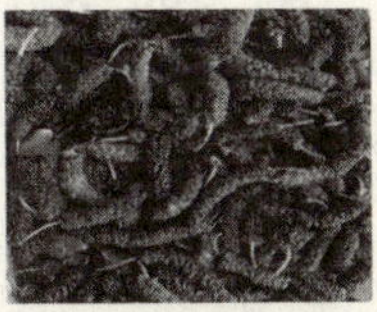	Mulberry (*shehtoot*): 1 *katori* (100 g) = 43 Cal
4. 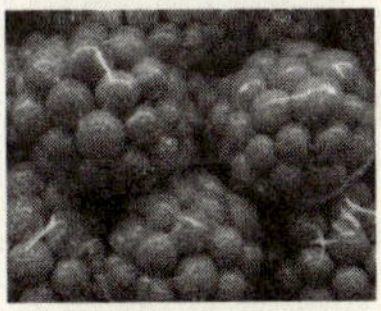	Raspberry (*rasabharee*): 1 *katori* (100 g) = 53 Cal
5. 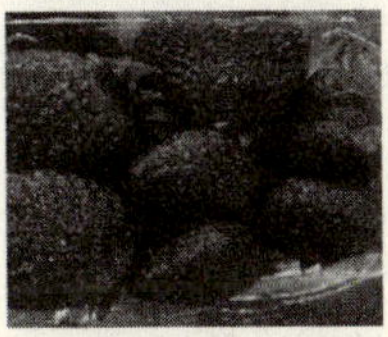	Strawberry (*stroberee*): 1 *katori* (100 g) = 33 Cal
6. 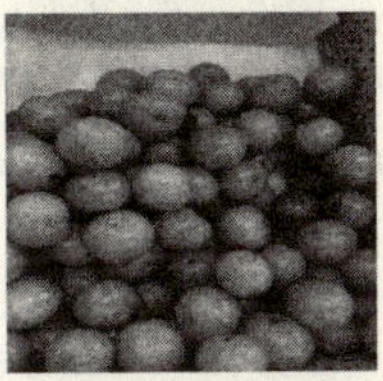	Indian gooseberry (*amla*): 1 *katori* (100 g) = 48 Cal
7. 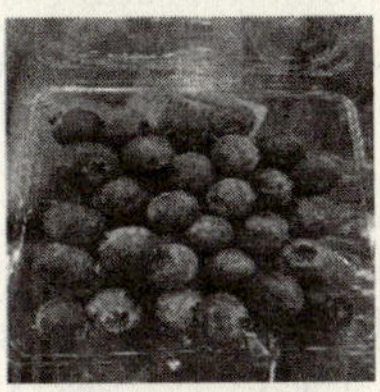	Blueberry (*blooberee/neelbadri*): 1 *katori* (100 g) = 57 Cal
8. 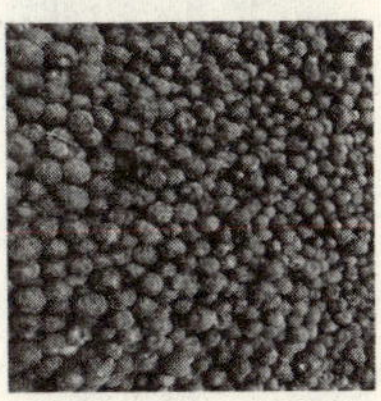	Sherbet berry (*phalsa*): 1 *katori* (100g) = 50 Cal

Source: Author's own compilation

Avocados

Avocado (*makhanphal*) is a large, berry-type fruit. It has become increasingly popular due to its nutritional properties, including healthy fats, fibre, vitamins and minerals..

Nutrition Facts

One 100 g serving of avocado provides 160 Cal, 8.5 g carbohydrates (0.7 g sugars, 6.7 g fibre), 2 g protein and 14.7 g fat (including 2.1 g saturated and 9.8 g monounsaturated fat). It is a rich source of vitamin E, vitamin K, potassium, phytosterols and carotenoids such as lutein and zeaxanthin (these values may vary depending on the source).

Popular Health-Centric Uses

Increasingly, avocados are recognised as healthy fruits, and consumption has increased in India as well.

Scientific Studies

1. High monounsaturated fats (MUFAs), fibre and phytosterols in avocados make it one of the healthiest food options.
2. The avocado oil is also healthy, consisting of 71 percent MUFAs, 13 percent polyunsaturated fats (PUFAs) and 16 percent saturated fatty acids.[131] Avocado oil is a high-heat stable oil used for cooking (frying, roasting and dressings), skincare and haircare.
3. Preliminary clinical studies show that avocado consumption may improve blood vessel health and inflammation.[132] A recent meta-analysis shows that it can marginally decrease cholesterol levels.[133]
4. In a six-month study of nearly 1,000 adults with belly fat, eating one avocado every day slightly improved healthy fat levels in the blood. People who didn't eat avocados showed changes in blood fats linked to more belly fat, higher blood sugar and worse cholesterol, but these changes weren't seen in the avocado group.[134]
5. Some other studies also suggest that avocados may support weight loss by increasing satiety and enhancing metabolism.[135]
6. Avocado intake has been shown to increase memory and cognition. However, these are preliminary trials.[136] [137]

Spices

Curcumin

Curcumin is the active ingredient present in turmeric (*haldi*).[138] Turmeric (*Curcuma longa*) is a type of herb belonging to the ginger family that is widely grown in the southern and southwestern tropical Asia region.

Nutrition Facts

Per 100 g, turmeric powder contains 60–70 percent carbohydrates, 6–8 percent protein, 5–10 percent fat and 2–7 percent dietary fibre. It also provides minerals and is especially valued for its phytochemicals, including curcuminoids and essential oils, which contribute to its colour, flavour and health benefits (these values may vary depending on the source).

Popular Health-Centric Uses

Haldi has long been used in the preparation of Ayurvedic drugs. It is said to have healing properties and is often applied on wounds for the acceleration of healing. Turmeric is also known to have been used for centuries in India and China for the medical treatment of illnesses such as dermatological diseases, infections (cold/cough), stress and depression.

Scientific Studies

1. There have been numerous research trials on *haldi* and curcumin, but few have shown clear results.
2. One positive result of curcumin is on Alzheimer's disease.[139] Indeed, it is often argued that the low incidence of Alzheimer's disease in India is due to the high intake of curcumin.
3. More research has been conducted on its possible anti-cancer activity.[140] [141]
4. Experimentally, wound healing and anti-inflammatory properties have been shown.[142]
5. Similarly, some studies have shown glucose-lowering and anti-inflammatory properties in diabetes.[143] [144]

6. A meta-analysis has shown that curcumin (especially nano preparation, along with piperine to enhance blood levels) can produce weight loss and decrease abdominal girth.[145]
7. Other uses include benefits in depression[146], liver fat[147] and repair of exercise-induced muscle damage.[148]

Curcumin by itself has poor bioavailability. It cannot be used in human beings in the same way as in animals, hence limiting its benefits. However, piperine in black pepper has been shown to increase its bioavailability by 2,000 percent. Some analogues of curcumin are being developed to enhance its effects.

Nano-turmeric

The clinical implication of native curcumin is hindered due to low solubility, physico-chemical instability, poor bioavailability, rapid metabolism and poor pharmacokinetics. Hence, researchers have attempted to enhance the biological and pharmacological activity of curcumin and overcome its drawbacks by developing efficient delivery systems, particularly nanoencapsulation. Research efforts so far and data from the available literature have shown a satisfactory potential of nano-range formulations of curcumin (nanocurcumin).[149]

How Can Turmeric Be Used?

Drink Golden Milk

Golden milk is an ancient Ayurvedic recipe that can be made in a number of ways. It is just turmeric paste mixed with warm milk. You can use skimmed milk for this recipe. To make the paste, simply bring ½ cup filtered water to a low simmer and then mix in ¼ cup of ground turmeric, stirring constantly until it makes a thick paste (this can take 5–10 minutes), adding more water as needed. To make the golden milk, mix ½ tsp of paste with 1 cup of milk in a saucepan and cook over medium-low heat for about 5 minutes. You can also add other spices like cinnamon, ginger or black pepper. Store the remaining turmeric paste in your fridge for two weeks. This is fabulous before bedtime!

Caution

A known safety issue with curcumin and/or turmeric is contamination with heavy metals – either due to turmeric grown on contaminated soil or due to intentional adulteration with, for example, lead chromate. Detailed discussion on safely aspects is available for reference.[150]

Cinnamon

Cinnamon (*dalchini*), the brown, mildly bitter and mildly spicy cooking herb, is popularly used in traditional Indian, Persian and Turkish cuisines as a flavouring agent in curries. Previously, it was believed to be beneficial for diabetes, which has now been proven in a research study published in an international journal by our group at NDOC and Fortis-CDOC Diabetes Hospital, New Delhi, India.[151]

Nutrition Facts

Per 100 g, cinnamon provides about 247 Cal, 80.6 g carbohydrates (including ~ 2.2 g sugars and ~ 53 g fibre), 4 g protein and 1.2 g fat. It is a very rich source of calcium and iron and also supplies vitamin K, vitamin E and manganese (these values may vary depending on the source).

Popular Health-Centric Uses

Cinnamon has been used as a health enhancer and digestive.

Scientific Studies

Scientific studies are few, and many of them are not strong enough to lead to conclusions.

1. Diabetes and lipids
   - i. In general, there has been some benefit in usage of cinnamon in patients with type 2 diabetes and lipid disorders.[152]
   - ii. A randomised and blinded trial with good design carried out by our group shows that the use of cinnamon:[151]
     - I. improves blood sugar control,
     - II. helps to reduce body weight and abdominal girth,

    III. reduces blood fats (lipids: triglycerides, total cholesterol, LDL cholesterol), and
    IV. helps in lowering blood pressure.
    V. It may have some effects on satiety.[153]
2. Other diseases: It may have some use in Alzheimer's disease[154] and alleviating post-menopausal symptoms.[155]

How to Use Cinnamon

1. Up to 2–3 g/day (½ tsp) can be consumed.
2. The commonly used forms of cinnamon for oral consumption:
    i. Fresh hand-ground cinnamon powder, ½ tsp, can be taken with ½ glass of water (150 ml). It can also be added to oatmeal, coffee, salads, meats, vegetable preparations, rice pudding, protein shakes and so on.
    ii. For non-diabetics, hand-ground cinnamon powder can be used along with honey/lime juice/orange juice.
3. Cinnamon should be avoided by:
    i. pregnant women,
    ii. lactating mothers,
    iii. patients taking blood-thinning medications,
    iv. children (below eighteen years of age) and
    v. people with significant liver damage.

Easy Reading 10

Cinnamon (*Dalchini*): A Metabolically Efficient Herb

A sixty-five-year-old lady with type 2 diabetes, heart disease and hypertension told me, 'Doc, I eat plenty of herbs and also cinnamon.' I encouraged her and told her that among these herbal compounds, cinnamon will work best for her. Then I explained the following in detail.

Cinnamon was originally cultivated in Sri Lanka and India. It is a brown, mildly bitter, mildly spicy cooking herb popularly used in traditional Indian, Persian and Turkish cuisines as a flavouring agent to curries. In Western countries, it is sprinkled on toast and lattes, and cinnamon rolls are popular.

Although many varieties exist, most commercial preparations are derived from *Cinnamomum cassia*. The aroma and flavour of cinnamon derive from its essential oil and principal component, cinnamaldehyde. Its use has been mentioned in the Bible and ancient Chinese tests. In Egyptian history, cinnamon was used to embalm mummies.

The composition of cinnamon is 11 percent water, 81 percent carbohydrates (including 53 percent dietary fibre), 4 percent protein and 1 percent fat. It is rich in calcium, iron, vitamin K and resins such as cinnamaldehyde, cinnamate, cinnamic acids and so on. Traditionally, a number of beneficial effects have been ascribed to cinnamon, including those on cough/cold, indigestion, hypertension, diabetes, memory, oral health, cancer and Alzheimer's disease. However, robust clinical trials and in-depth analysis are only available for some of these ailments, most importantly for diabetes and metabolic disorders.

In 2017, our group carried out a path-breaking robust scientific study (randomised controlled trial) of cinnamon in India. In this trial, 3 g cinnamon was given as capsules to fifty-eight people with metabolic syndrome (a condition when abdominal obesity, elevated blood sugar and deranged cholesterol and triglyceride levels occur together in the same individual). They were compared to another fifty-eight individuals with metabolic syndrome who did not receive cinnamon. The trial was conducted over a period of four months. When the results were analysed, we were pleasantly surprised. The use of cinnamon leads to a decrease in blood glucose, abdominal fat, weight, blood pressure and cholesterol levels. At the end of the study, many people had normal blood sugar, lipids and waist circumference, meaning thereby that, in them, metabolic syndrome no longer existed. This trial was widely appreciated by the scientific community, and since then, cinnamon use became popular in many patients of diabetes in India.[151]

Before and after our study, several other trials have been performed with cinnamon worldwide, and barring a few, most show a good effect on blood sugar and lipid levels. While results of these trials are clearly encouraging, longer trials are warranted. Cinnamon has also been used in patients with nasal allergies, HIV and COVID-19, but results are uncertain. It has been used in patients with IBS, though firm data is not available.

The metabolic action of cinnamon has been ascribed to multiple mechanisms. The polyphenol-rich cinnamon is a potential source of natural antioxidants, exhibiting strong scavenging (cleaning) properties for toxic material in cells, which may reduce stress (oxidative) on cellular functions. It facilitates the movement of cellular vehicles transporting glucose in the cells ('glucose transporters'), thus making its metabolism efficient. Additionally, it may delay the absorption of glucose after meals.

Per day, 2 to 3 g (½ tsp) of cinnamon intake has been shown to be safe. It can be taken as fresh hand-ground cinnamon powder: ½ tsp in half a glass of water (150 ml). It is advisable not to exceed intake of more than 5 g (1 tsp/day). It can also be added to oatmeal, tea, coffee, salads, meats, vegetable preparations, rice pudding, protein shakes and the like. For non-diabetic individuals, hand-ground cinnamon powder can be used along with honey/lime juice/orange juice. For patients with diabetes, it can be mixed with lime water and taken as such. It should be avoided in pregnant and lactating mothers, patients taking blood-thinning medications (anticoagulants called coumarins) and children/adolescents below eighteen years of age. People with significant liver damage should avoid cinnamon.

So once again, I told my patient, 'You can use other herbs used in cooking, but cinnamon is your showstopper.'

Note: This article, originally featured in *The Indian Express*, has been revised and updated from its initial published version.

Nuts and Dried Fruits

Nuts

Nuts are edible seeds, many of them encased in a hard shell. There are several types of nuts available. These nuts are usually consumed as snacks.

Nutrition Facts

Nuts have been increasingly researched for their nutritional properties. The following is a summary of their nutritional properties:

1. Nuts are rich in fibre, which results in the following benefits:
   i. Slow absorption of macronutrients
   ii. Increased production of good fatty acids (short-chain fatty acids), which decreases liver sugar production and increases good hormones (glucagon-like peptide-1), which, in turn, increases efficiency of glucose metabolism
2. Nuts have low carbohydrates and, hence, low GI.
3. They have a high content of beneficial fatty acids (MUFAs and PUFAs; see Chapter 2).
4. Nuts have a high content of magnesium.
5. In general, nuts have very high antioxidant capacity.

Popular Health-Centric Uses

In India, nuts are generally considered as healthy but with the following misconceptions:

1. Nuts are 'hot by nature' and should be avoided in hot weather.
2. Eating nuts will make you gain weight.

Both are not true. An increasing number of studies show that consumption of nuts within prescribed calories is healthy.

Scientific Studies

There are numerous studies done worldwide. In diabetes, nuts have been extensively researched by our group, showing many of the benefits listed next. We have shown that nuts are excellent snacks for patients with diabetes.

1. Several studies show an inverse association between nut consumption and diabetes (both for prevention and management) and cardiovascular disease. Nuts also decrease cholesterol levels and protect the heart. Intake of nuts, along with a prescribed calorie plan for any individual, decreases body and abdominal fat and, to some extent, fat in the liver.[156 157 158 159 160]

2. The benefits on post-meal blood sugar are evident when nuts (pistachios [*pista*], almonds [*badam*] and the like) are taken alone or with high-carb foods. Our studies show that nuts taken before meals lower postprandial blood glucose levels.[161 162]
3. Nuts may also delay decline in cognitive dysfunction as in Alzheimer's disease.[163]
4. Some reviews suggest that nut consumption also increases longevity and prevents death.[164]
5. In a well-conducted trial, it has been shown that including nuts in a regular diet significantly improved auto-reported orgasmic function and sexual desire.[165]

TABLE 5.6 Calorie and Fat Content of Various Nuts Available in India

Variety of Nut	Calorie (Single Nut)	Calorie (1 oz Nuts)	Total Fat (g/100 g Raw Nut)	Saturated Fat (g/100 g Raw Nut)	MUFA (g/100 g Raw Nut)	PUFA (g/100 g Raw Nut)
Almonds (*badam*)	7.7	166	49	4.3	32	12
Cashews (*kaju*)	9	163	46	7.8	28	8
Peanuts (*moongphali*)	5.9	166	49	8.1	24	16
Pistachios (*pista*)	4	172	45	4.0	23	13
Walnuts (*akhrot*)	13	182	65	5.2	9	47

Note: MUFA: Monounsaturated fat; PUFA: Polyunsaturated fat
Sources: Data from Hernández-Alonso *et al.*[166] and Longvah *et al.*[5]
Any differences in nutrient values reflect variations in data sources, analytical methods and preparation methods.

The following are other points not included in Table 5.6.

1. Almonds are the richest in vitamin E and fibre.
2. Pistachios contain the highest levels of beta-carotene and lutein-zeaxanthin, with high fibre content (second only to almonds).
3. All nuts are good sources of dietary fibre.

Dried Fruits

Dried fruits are a concentrated form of fruit (part or whole) with low moisture content—for example, apricots (*khubani*), berries, grapes (*angoor*), kiwifruit (*kiwi*), mangoes (*aam*), papayas (*papita*) and bananas (*kela*). In dried forms, these are easier to store.

Nutrition Facts

1. In contrast to nuts, dried fruits are mainly composed of carbohydrates (60–70 percent) with low content of protein and fat and a good amount of fibre.
2. Some dried fruits, blueberries, cranberries (*karonda*), cherries, strawberries (*stroberee*) and mangoes are commonly infused with different types of sugar solution (or fruit juice) concentrate before drying and should not be included in this category.
3. Some contain a good amount of fructose (for example, raisins [*kishmish*], figs [*anjeer*], dates [*khajoor*], which may explain their relatively good GI.
4. Dried fruits have high antioxidant properties, and sun drying enhances them.
5. Sun-dried raisins contain antioxidants, phytochemicals (more concentrated than in grapes) and resveratrol.
6. Beta-carotene is highest in apricots (*sookhi khubani*), followed by peaches and prunes (*sookha aaloo bukhara*).
7. Most contain a high amount of potassium.

Popular Health-Centric Uses

Generally, there is confusion whether dried fruits are healthy or not. For example, raisins (*kishmish*) are often considered to be bad for patients with diabetes.

TABLE 5.7 Calorie, Carbohydrate and Fibre Content of Various Dried Fruits *(Sookhe Meve)*

Variety of Dried Fruit	Calories	Carbohydrates (g)	Fibre (g)
Dates (*khajoor*)	282	75	8
Raisins (*kishmish*)	299	79	3.7
Figs (*anjeer*)	249	64	9.8
Apricots (*sookhi khubani*)	241	63	7.2
Prunes (*sookha aaloo bukhara*)	240	64	7.1

Note: All values are per 100 g portion.
Source: Author's own compilation
Any differences in nutrient values reflect variations in data sources, analytical methods and preparation methods.

Scientific Studies

1. In general, dried fruits are healthier than fresh fruits.[166] Raisins are rich in fibre, potassium and antioxidants with a low to moderate glycaemic and insulinemic index.[167]
2. Studies show they can reduce blood pressure and improve cholesterol and triglyceride (blood fats), thus benefiting heart health.[167]
3. Intake of dried fruits within an overall healthy diet plan may decrease weight and benefit fat in liver.
4. Raisins (*kishmish*) may be beneficial for blood sugar level, help insulin secretion and decrease blood pressure.[168 169]

Overall, small amounts of dried fruits and raisins are healthy dietary options and may even be suitable for people with type 2 diabetes (see Easy Reading 11). Excess consumption should be avoided.

Easy Reading 11

Dates (*Khajoor*) and Other Dried Fruits (*Sookhe Meve*): Are They Fine for Patients with Diabetes and/or Obesity?

An Indian with diabetes has been living in Saudi Arabia and comes to me for a check-up from time to time. This time, he asked me, 'Doc, dates are very popular there. Can I eat them? I hope my glucose levels will not be disturbed.'

Another patient, a seventy-year-old lady, said, 'Doc I am guilty of eating raisins every day. I think it is going to increase my blood sugar. What is to be done?'

I reassured them and explained to them in simple words the following facts.

What Are Dried Fruits?

A concentrated form of fresh fruits with low moisture content is known as dried fruits. These include whole fruits (berries and grapes [*angoor*]) or half/slices of fruits (*kiwi*s, mangoes). The dried form of fruits permits long shelf life and availability.

Apples (*seb*), apricots (*khubani*), currants, dates (*khajoor*), figs (*anjeer*), peaches (*aadu*), pears (*nashpati*), prunes (*sookha aaloo bukhara*) and raisins (*kishmish*) are popular dried fruits.

Several bioactive compounds are found in dried fruits: vitamins, minerals, carotenoids and phytosterols. All these are needed for good health. Sun-dried raisins (*kishmish*) retain the minerals and most of the phytochemicals, antioxidants and resveratrol of the grapes. Interestingly, sun-drying enhances the antioxidant content of raisins. Dried fruits contain about two-thirds carbohydrates with low protein content and a high amount of fibre.

Effects of Dried Fruits on Health

Indians have a tradition of eating nuts and raisins. These are popularly given on festivals and weddings as gifts.

Among all dried fruits, grapes have been investigated the most. It has been shown that seeds or powder of skin of grapes could improve inflammation and insulin secretion, two key metabolic indicators of good health. Raisins have been shown to increase powerful metabolically active hormones (for example, glucagon-like peptide-1), which have a good effect on the pancreas. Longer clinical studies, although few, show similar data. Overall, a limited number of raisins incorporated in healthy diets is not likely to increase blood sugar values and may be beneficial.

Date fruits are popular throughout the Middle Eastern countries. There are various stages of dates. The *Tamer* stage is the maturation stage where the date fruit is dried, firm and dark in colour. This is widely available in Indian markets. These can be eaten as snacks or with meals. A variety of dates are available, and some have lower effects on glucose than other varieties. Some good trials show that intake of dates does not have a significant effect on blood glucose, cholesterol, body weight and blood pressure. Again, contrary to popular opinion, small amounts of dates are not going to cause any harm in patients with diabetes and/or obesity.

Should a Patient with Diabetes Eat Dried Fruits?

The available data shows that a limited quantity of dried fruits taken regularly does not affect blood sugar or body weight. However, there are not many studies, and we need long-term data. Further, if somebody does not follow a healthy lifestyle, including healthy foods and daily exercise, and takes large amounts of dates, raisins and other dried fruits over the usual calorie intake, he/she will have weight gain, and some impact on blood sugar is a likely possibility.

So a Bedouin who is walking miles daily can eat plenty of dates and probably nothing may happen to his health parameters. If a 'couch potato' does that, he/she may have bad consequences. So moderate intake of raisins (in combination with nuts, *kaju-kishmish*) and dates is fine for an active and fit person with or without diabetes.

Note: This article, originally featured in *The Indian Express*, has been revised and updated from its initial published version.

Milk and Dairy Products

1. Milk is a white-coloured liquid nutrient mostly derived from the mammary gland of mammals. It is divided into dairy milk and non-dairy milk (for example, almond [*badam*] milk, coconut milk, rice milk and soy milk). Milk is processed into a variety of products such as cream, butter (*makhan*), yoghurt (*dahi*), ice cream and cheese.
2. Pasteurised milk: When all pathogens are destroyed by treatment with mild heat, milk is pasteurised.
3. Fermented milk: Left standing, milk turns sour because of the effect of lactic acid formed by bacteria. Such products (sour cream, buttermilk [*chaach*] and so on) are believed to be good for digestion.
4. Organic milk: Normal milk may contain some residue of antibiotics that cows were treated with, while organic milk is obtained from cows not treated with antibiotics. Organic

milk may contain higher amounts of omega-3 PUFAs, conjugated linoleic acid, α-tocopherol and iron than normal cow milk.

5. A2 milk: There are thirteen genetic variants of β-casein found in cow's milk. The A1 and A2 variants of beta-casein differ at amino acid position 67 with histidine in A1 and proline in A2 milk as a result of a single nucleotide difference. Both A1 and A2 varieties offer the same nutrient content. However, for some people, drinking cow's milk with A1 casein can cause abdominal discomfort due to the release of certain peptides (BCM7) that are produced when this protein is digested. No positive effects were found for cardiovascular markers with A2 milk.[170] Overall, A2 milk is not superior to regular milk in nutrition or cardiovascular outcomes and is mainly useful for people who have difficulty digesting standard milk.
6. Soya milk: Also known as soy milk, it is a plant-based alternative to cow's milk made from soybeans. It is produced by soaking soybeans in water, grinding them, boiling the mixture and then filtering out the solids. Soy milk has gained popularity as a dairy-free alternative for individuals who are lactose-intolerant, allergic to dairy proteins or following a vegan diet. It may offer benefits to adults with blood lipids, blood pressure and inflammation; however, more data is needed.[171]

Nutrition Facts

1. Milk is the richest, most appropriate source of nutrition for children and adults. Nutrition composition of various types of milk is given in Table 5.8.
2. Among proteins, it contains casein and whey proteins.
3. Milk contains lactose, glucose and galactose as the main varieties of carbohydrates. Lactose (consisting of glucose and galactose) is the main carbohydrate.

Milk and Milk Products and Health

Milk is an excellent food but not perfect. There is a general misconception that avoidance of milk will be beneficial for diabetes and obesity.

1. Milk promotes growth velocity and greater attainment of height in children.
2. In general, in low-income countries like India, where poor diet quality is prevalent, intake of milk could improve health. This is not the case with both people who have better diet quality in India (high socio-economic stratum) and in developed countries.
3. Conjugated linoleic acid in milk may help in decreasing body fat and may have other health-promoting properties, but more data is needed.
4. Insulin-like growth factors are found in milk in limited quantities. However, a higher amount has been seen in milk of cows that have been treated with chemicals (growth factors). These insulin-like growth factors have been implicated in the increased risk of some cancers (described later).
5. About three cups (450 ml) of milk is adequate consumption for an adult.

Bone Health/Fractures

1. Milk and other dairy products may diminish the risk of hip fracture.[172]
2. There is some evidence that higher yoghurt consumption was associated with reduced hip fracture risk.[173]

Obesity

1. No overall effects of milk intake are seen on body weight.[174]
2. The effects of milk, low-fat milk and cheese were similar.
3. Results in children are uncertain, and some studies show that higher milk fat is associated with lower obesity, but more research is needed.[175]
4. Yoghurt consumption may be related to some weight loss.[176]

Blood Pressure, Blood Cholesterol and Heart Disease

1. It is believed that the potassium content of milk may decrease blood pressure. However, this point has not been proven.
2. Milk or milk products (up to 200 g/day) have not been associated with occurrence of heart disease and strokes,

though the evidence is not conclusive and may depend on the type of dairy product.[177]

3. Cheese intake may have moderate benefits for heart disease and mortality.[178]
4. Milk and cheese may have some beneficial effects on stroke.[179]

Diabetes

Type 1 Diabetes

1. Since cow milk protein has some similarities with pancreatic insulin-producing cells, it has been shown that these can harm the pancreas and cause type 1 (juvenile) diabetes.[180] Although this idea is immensely popular and often debated, it has not been conclusively proven.

Type 2 Diabetes

1. Dairy consumption is associated with no increased risk or slightly lower risk of type 2 diabetes.[181] The risk reduction is particularly evident when milk is compared with sugar-sweetened beverages (SSBs) and fruit juices.

Cancer

1. In well-conducted studies, milk consumption is associated with a higher risk of prostate cancer.[182]
2. On the other hand, studies about its effect on breast, ovarian and other cancers yield mixed results. However, there is possibly an increased risk of endometrial cancer but reduced risk of colorectal cancer.[174]

Lactose Intolerance

1. Some people lack lactose, the enzyme that breaks down lactose in the intestine. If milk is consumed by these people, it causes bloating, gaseous distension of the abdomen, diarrhoea and abdominal pain.[183]
2. Lactose intolerance in most people is genetically determined, but for some, it follows intestinal infections.
3. To overcome this, lactose-free alternatives such as soy milk, lactose-free cow's milk and cheese have become available.

Objections/Myths Regarding Milk Intake

1. Pure lacto-vegetarians do not like to consume milk. This form of diet is followed by Hindu and Jain religious communities.
2. Concern about health of animals (keeping cows pregnant, killing of all male offspring and so on) may also cause people to avoid milk.
3. There is a fear of increased risk of diabetes and acne.

Pertinent Points from Table 5.8

1. Buffalo, sheep and yak milk have the highest calorie and fat content.
2. Buffalo and almond milk have the highest calcium content, while soy milk has the lowest.

Curd and Yoghurt

Both curd and yoghurt are termed *dahi* in Hindi, although both differ, as explained below.

1. Curd (*dahi*) is made from bacterial fermentation of milk.
2. To make curd, usually cultures of friendly bacteria such as Lactobacillus are used.
3. *Dahi* is made by curdling the milk with acidic lemon juice or vinegar. It contains *Lactobacillus* bacterium, that is, lactic acid bacteria. *Dahi* is mostly made at home.
4. For making yoghurt, *Lactobacillus bulgaricus* and *Streptococcus thermophiles* cultures are used. It is an industrial product. Yoghurt is available commercially in various flavours.

Nutrition Facts

1. Plain yoghurt contains, per 100 g, 97 Cal, 3.98 g carbohydrates, 9 g protein and 5 g fat. It also has a good amount of vitamin B and some calcium (these values may vary depending on the source).
2. Sweetened and other modified commercial yoghurts may contain a high amount of sugar. *Misti doi* is a sweetened yoghurt popular in Bengal.
3. Strained yoghurt (a thicker variety of yoghurt obtained after passing it through thin cloth to remove whey protein) mixed with other ingredients is sold as *srikhand* in India.
4. Probiotic yoghurt has extra *Lactobacillus* bacteria added to it.

TABLE 5.8 Nutritional Composition of Various Types of Milk

Type of Milk	Water Content (%)	Calorie Content (Cal)	Protein Content (%)	Lactose Content (%)	Fat Content (%)	Saturated Fat (%)	Casein-to-Whey Protein Ratio	Calcium (mg/ 100 ml)	Phosphorus (mg/ 100 ml)
Cow	87.80	72.8	3.32–3.49	4.42–4.76	4.68–4.88	2.70	80:20	120.24	88.08
Buffalo	83.18	107	3.87–4.48	4.70–4.86	6.38–8.30	4.63	80:20	178.59	109.22
Sheep	82	108	4.50–6.60	3.90–4.90	6.99	4.54	80:20	--	--
Goat	83.20	69	3.42	4.16	3.84	2.66	80:20	129.08	98.91
Camel (milk obtained from *Anand/Khera*)	86.50	66.5	3.00	4.25	4.43	2.4	76:24	--	--
Camel (milk obtained from *Kutchh*)	86.50	66.5	2.66	3.77	2.90	2.4	76:24	--	--
Yak	--	--	5.10	4.40	6.50	3.90	80:20	131	106
Reduced fat (2% fat) cow	89.33	50	3.30	5.01	1.97	1.25	--	117	94
Low fat (1% fat) cow	89.92	42	3.37	5.20	0.97	0.63	--	119	95
Skimmed milk	90.84	34	3.37	5.09	0.08	0.11	--	125	101
Soy milk	88.05	54	3.27	6.28 (carbs)	1.75	0.20	--	25	52
Almond milk	96.54	15	0.40	1.31 (carbohydrate)	0.96	0.08	--	184	9

Source: Author's own compilation and based on data from Yoganandi *et al.*,[184] Kapadiya *et al.*,[185] Mohapatra *et al.*,[186] Nikkhah,[187 188] Longvah *et al.*,[5] Singh *et al.*,[189] US Department of Agriculture,[190 191 192] Skeaff *et al.*,[193] Rafiq *et al.*,[194] Shamsia.[195]
Any differences in nutrient values reflect variations in data sources, analytical methods and preparation methods.

Scientific Studies

1. Effect on the intestinal system:
   i. Yoghurt consumption has the potential to improve gut health. It can reduce inflammation by enhancing immunity and intestinal barrier functions. It has some effects on regulating appetite.
   ii. It may hasten recovery from diarrhoea and help non-specific abdominal distress. Its role in diarrhoea associated with antibiotics usage has been researched without any conclusions.
2. Other health effects:
   i. Yoghurt intake has been shown to improve the action of insulin in the body and decrease harmful liver fat. For these actions, it is better than milk.[196] It may reduce body fat and cause some weight loss.
   ii. Recently, the Food and Drug Administration, USA, has cleared yoghurt for possible benefits on type 2 diabetes as per evidence.[197] FDA has concluded that there is limited information supporting this claim. In other words, eating yoghurt regularly, at least two cups (three servings) per week, may reduce the risk of type 2 diabetes according to limited scientific evidence.[198]
   iii. Intake of yoghurt has been shown to increase bone strength and thus has the potential to decrease fracture risk in some studies.[173]

Cheese

Cheese is the solidified product of milk and protein (coagulated casein). Varieties depend on the source of milk and flavouring with herbs, spices and wood smoke.

Nutrition Facts

1. There are various kinds of cheese.
   i. Swiss (yellow cheese harder than butter [*makhan*], originating from Switzerland)
   ii. Feta (brittle cheese from sheep milk, from Greece)
   iii. Cheddar (hard yellow to orange, from the United Kingdom)

iv. Mozzarella (made from buffalo or cow's milk, from Italy)
v. Cottage (*paneer,* white, of rubbery consistency, from India)

2. These have different contents of nutrients per 100 g: 1.3–5.4 g carbs, 21–29 g fats and 14–27 g protein. Cheese is rich in calcium and vitamin B_{12}.
3. Most types of cheese are gluten-free.

Scientific Studies

1. Health concerns have been raised because of high amounts of saturated fatty acids and salt in cheese.
2. Intake of cheese could increase the feeling of fullness and satiety.
3. Overall, beneficial effects of cheese intake on heart disease have been seen.[199]
4. In addition, no increased effect on mortality (death rate) has been observed.
5. Consumption of cheese may decrease the risk of stroke.[179]
6. Cheese intake is reported to be associated with a lower risk of hip fractures.[200]

Cottage Cheese

1. Cottage cheese (*paneer*) is a popular indigenous product that is obtained by heat treating the milk followed by acid coagulation using suitable acids like citric acid, lactic acid, tartaric acid, alum or sour whey. The whey formed is removed to some extent through filtration and pressing.
2. *Paneer* represents one of the soft varieties of the cheese family and is used in culinary dishes or snacks.

Nutrition Facts

One serving of 100 g cottage cheese from cow milk (5 percent fat) contains 265 Cal energy, 1.2 g carbs, 24.2 g fat, 8 g protein and 208 mg calcium. *Paneer*'s fat and protein content can vary depending on the milk type and preparation method. Buffalo milk or full-fat cow's milk *paneer* has higher fat, while protein typically ranges from 18–21 g per 100 g (these values may vary depending on the source).

Popular Health-Centric Uses

1. *Paneer* is well known for being a healthy vegetarian food because it is rich in protein and calcium.
2. Also, it is popularly used for bone health and development in children and reduction of fracture risk.
3. Despite the established benefits, some people avoid dairy in their diet due to a belief that it is detrimental to health, especially in those with osteoarthritis and rheumatoid arthritis.
4. Further, some avoid dairy products believing that it may increase blood glucose levels in patients with diabetes. However, there is no evidence that such people could benefit by avoiding dairy consumption.

Scientific Studies

1. Consumption of cottage cheese as a snack leads to a similar metabolic response to liquid protein.[201]
2. Also, research shows that cottage cheese has the same satiating power as eggs, making it a protein-rich option for appetite control.[202]
3. Evidence suggests consumption of dairy products reduces body fat but not necessarily body weight due to a preservation of lean body mass.

How Can Cottage Cheese Be Used?

Cottage cheese can be eaten as scrambled cottage cheese (*paneer bhurji*) or other paneer preparations as a part of Indian cuisine. It can be grilled or used as a filling in *besan cheela* sandwiches or as a topping on pizza.

Easy Reading 12

The Good and Not-So-Good Sides of Vegetarian Diets

A sixty-five-year-old frail-looking man with diabetes and weak muscles asked me, 'Doc, I am following non-veg diets. People say vegetarian diets are better.' Another patient (fifty-six-year-old female) with diabetes, deranged kidney functions and a family history of colon cancer asked, 'Doc, can I switch over from vegetarian to non-vegetarian diets?' After the following discussion, I will state my answers based on evidence.

Vegetarian diets are becoming increasingly popular in countries that are predominantly non-vegetarian. The reasons are endorsement by celebrities and protective sentiments for animals. Vegetarian diets, although lumped under a single name, are heterogenous. Lacto-vegetarian diets exclude meat, fish, poultry and eggs as well as foods that contain them and include dairy products (milk, cheese, yoghurt [*dahi*] and butter [*makhan*]). Ovo-vegetarian diets allow eggs but exclude meat, poultry, seafood and dairy products. Lacto-ovo vegetarian diets allow dairy products and eggs and exclude meat, fish and poultry. Finally, vegan diets exclude meat, poultry, fish, eggs and dairy products and foods that contain these products (see Chapter 3). Most Indians are lacto-ovo vegetarians. The essence and goodness of vegetarian diets are in the consumption of plants, nuts, legumes and fruits.

Plant-Based Vegetarian Diets Are Good!

Following a 'good' vegetarian diet has multiple benefits. This diet decreases the risk of heart disease and lowers blood cholesterol and weight. In addition, intestinal diseases (diverticulitis), kidney stones, kidney dysfunction, cataracts and possibly some cancers are lower in those who follow vegetarian/vegan diets. Curiously, these diets do not decrease the risk of strokes and may even increase it. Even short-term (up to three months) following of vegan diets may decrease blood sugar levels in a patient with type 2 diabetes. Pulses (*dalen*), soy (*soya*), nuts/dried fruits (*meve/sookhe meve*), seeds (*beej*), chickpeas (*chane*), kidney beans (*rajma*), black gram (*urad dal*), green gram (*moong dal*), pigeon peas (*arhar/toor dal*), lentils (*masoor dal*), etc. are important sources of plant proteins. These are generally low in saturated fat and provide fibre and phytochemicals, whereas animal proteins from meat (*maans*), eggs (*ande*) and dairy (*doodh aur dugdh utpadan*) are richer in essential amino acids but often higher in saturated fat and cholesterol. Higher intake of plant proteins is associated with lower risk of type 2 diabetes, obesity and cardiovascular disease, while excessive reliance on animal proteins may increase cardiometabolic risk.

Then Why Do Many Vegetarian Indians Have Diabetes, Heart and Liver Disease?

Just following a 'vegetarian diet' is not good enough. Ingredients have to be balanced and should be conducive to metabolism. There are two major issues in Indian vegetarian diets. First, there is a high intake of refined carbohydrates (rice, *naan* and so on) in major meals. This majorly upsets all metabolic elements (sugar, triglycerides and the like) post meals. Second, there is a high intake of saturated fat/trans-fats (*ghee*, butter, high-fat milk, coconut oil, oils derived from palm, partially hydrogenated vegetable oils and so on), which get deposited in thick layers in the liver and arteries, prevent smooth functioning of cells and blood circulation, and even block it. Besides other problems, these two issues alone can lead to diabetes, heart and liver disease.

Downsides of Vegetarian Diets and What Can We Do about It?

Several deficiencies may occur with prolonged vegetarian diets. These deficiencies include that of vitamin B_{12}, which is primarily obtained from non-vegetarian diets. Its deficiency can cause nerve damage, which is also prevalent in diabetes. So patients with diabetes who are vegetarians should get their B_{12} levels checked, if possible. If it is low or they are on a drug called metformin, then supplementation with this vitamin is warranted.

There is a possibility of deficiency of iron, zinc, calcium (especially in those who do not take dairy) and omega-3 PUFAs (primarily derived from fish). The latter is essential for nerves and blood triglycerides. To some extent, it can be supplemented by using canola and soy oils in cooking and walnuts (*akhrot*), ground flaxseed (*alsi*) and soybeans, but more is required. Some sources of iron include beans (*phaliyan* such as *sem* and *rajma*), dark-green leafy vegetables, peas (*matar*), lentils (*dal*), enriched cereals (*poshan-yukt anaj*) and dried fruits (*sookhe meve*). However, iron absorption from plant sources is inefficient. For better absorption of iron, foods rich in vitamin C are needed, such as citrus (orange [*santra*], sweet lime [*mausambi*], tomatoes [*tamatar*], cabbage [*patta gobhi*] and broccoli [*brokolee*]), to be taken at the time that iron-containing foods are being eaten. Zinc is essential for survival of cells and builds immunity. Like iron, it is poorly absorbed from vegetarian diets. Eating cheese, whole grains, soy products, legumes (*sabut dal*) and nuts could improve zinc status in the body. Vegans may be at risk for iodine deficiency and may even develop a goitre. Iodine can be obtained from iodised salt and also from dairy, eggs and some yoghurts (*dahi*). Finally, because of absence of dairy in vegan/similar diets, these people are prone to weakening of bones and fractures.

Importantly, vegetarians are short of high-quality protein, especially if they do not take eggs and dairy products. In many Indians whose muscles are weak ('sarcopenia'), this further causes low muscle functions and weakness, increases risk of several diseases and also affects bones. In selected individuals, especially older vegetarians whose food intake is low, protein supplementation is required. Good sources of protein include soybeans, lentils, cowpeas, peanuts (*moongphali*), almonds (*badam*), Bengal gram, flax seeds, oats (*jai*) and pumpkin seeds (*kaddu ke beej*).

My Answers to the Patients

My answer to the sixty-five-year-old frail-looking man with diabetes and weak muscles is that he should not leave non-vegetarian diets because these are good sources of protein, and additionally, he should add good vegetarian sources of protein. This will benefit his muscles and bones. Second, I replied to the fifty-six-year-old female to continue with a vegetarian diet and adjust protein intake (with the help of a nutritionist) according to kidney functions. I discussed that she should avoid non-vegetarian foods, especially red meat, which has been linked to colon cancer.

A balanced vegetarian diet will do wonders for health and metabolism, provided it does not contain a dirty bag of refined carbs and saturated fats and care is taken to avoid possible deficiencies of vitamins and minerals.

Note: This article, originally featured in *The Indian Express*, has been revised and updated from its initial published version.

Dietary Cholesterol

Cholesterol content of various foods is listed further in Table 5.9.

Eggs

Chicken eggs are a staple breakfast food.

Nutrition Facts

One large egg (50 g) provides about 72–78 Cal, negligible carbohydrates and no fibre. It has approximately 5 g fat, 186 mg cholesterol and 6 g protein and small amounts of vitamin D, vitamin A, and B-complex vitamins (these values may vary depending on the source).

Popular Health-Centric Uses

1. Generally, eggs are perceived as a good source of protein and nutrients.
2. However, many people avoid them as they are afraid that eating eggs will increase blood cholesterol (see discussion later).
3. Egg intake does not increase the likelihood of kidney disease if taken with a reasonable diet plan.

Other Sources of Dietary Cholesterol

Sausages, bacon, shellfish, butter (*makhan*), organ meats and, in India, saturated fat-laden oils, *ghee* and coconut oil are some sources of cholesterol. In the context of dairy products, it is found in dairy products that come from animal milk, such as whole milk, cheese, butter, *ghee*, cream and yoghurt. The amount varies, with higher levels in full-fat and processed dairy compared to low-fat or skimmed varieties.[203]

Blood Cholesterol and Eggs: Controversies and Guidelines

Limits for Dietary Cholesterol

1. Previously, dietary guidelines limited the permitted dietary cholesterol to less than 300 mg/day. Patients frequently tell me that they eat eggs but only the 'white part' and that will keep them 'safe' from heart disease. Dietary cholesterol, thus, has been demonised for decades in science and by the public. Most of the cholesterol from diets comes from the following items: eggs, sausages, bacon, shellfish, butter and organ meats. In India, it comes from whole-fat milk, cheese, saturated fat–laden oils, *ghee* and coconut oil. Indian diets, while mostly vegetarian, contain many of these items.
2. Guidelines for dietary cholesterol (less than 300 mg/day) were changed in 2013. At this time, the American Heart Association/American College of Cardiology advisory put no upper limits for dietary cholesterol. Further, the 2015 Dietary Guidelines Advisory Committee (in the US) stated that there was no appreciable relationship between dietary cholesterol intake and serum cholesterol levels. However, two recent US-based guidelines suggested caution and advised restrictions in dietary cholesterol intake, especially in patients with high cholesterol levels (summarised by Misra[204]).
3. A dietary recommendation in 2011 for Asian Indians (India) stated that dietary cholesterol should be taken in limited amount (200–300 mg/day) for healthy living and prevention of metabolic disorders.[205]

Nutrition Qualities of Eggs and Blood Cholesterol

1. Nutrition qualities: approximately 76 percent water, 12.6 percent protein, 9.5 percent fat and 0.7 percent carbohydrates. Proteins are split between the yolk and

the white, while fats are concentrated in the yolk. Eggs are rich in micronutrients such as vitamins A, D, E, K, B-group; minerals (phosphorus, selenium, iron, zinc); and choline. Lipids are predominantly unsaturated. Their lipids are predominantly unsaturated, with the yolk particularly rich in essential fatty acids like linoleic acid. Cholesterol is present at approximately 400 mg per 100 g.[206]

2. Eggs remain a major point of discussion while considering cholesterol in diets. Eggs contribute to about 25 percent of dietary cholesterol intake in the United States of America.[207] The annual per capita egg consumption also varies in India according to habitat. Consumption is more in urban areas than in rural areas.[208]
3. Egg yolk fats are packed into special particles made of triglycerides, cholesteryl esters, phospholipids, cholesterol and proteins. Eggs have more healthy unsaturated fats than saturated fats, and they also contain essential fats like linoleic acid. Eggs are high in cholesterol, but research shows they don't raise blood cholesterol in most healthy people. The effect depends more on saturated fat intake. Certain saturated fats (like myristic acid) raise cholesterol, while some unsaturated fats (like linoleic acid) lower it—eggs have very little myristic acid and much more linoleic acid. Overall, eggs are generally safe for the heart in healthy people, but 15–25 percent of people ('hyper-responders') may experience higher cholesterol with high egg intake.[206]
4. However, a study shows that among US adults, higher consumption of dietary cholesterol/eggs was significantly associated with a higher risk of incident heart disease and death.[209]
5. Egg consumption may be more harmful in patients with established and severe heart disease and heart failure.[204]

Indians and Blood Cholesterol

1. The average level of serum cholesterol is rising in the Indian population. About one-fourth of the population has high total cholesterol (higher than 200 mg/dL), and half have high LDL cholesterol (higher than 100 mg/dL) levels.

2. Interestingly, the highest average cholesterol levels were found in southern states (except one) and were mostly linked to development (average cholesterol levels in mg/dL: Kerala, 197; Goa, 196; Himachal, 185; Odisha, 176 and Karnataka, 175).[204]
3. Lipid abnormalities (high triglycerides, low HDL [good cholesterol] and high total cholesterol) lead to high risk of heart disease in Indians.

Healthy Diets and Blood Cholesterol

1. In developing countries, diets are progressively getting imbalanced with higher intake of calorie- and saturated fat-dense fast foods. As emphasised, cholesterol is high in most foods with high saturated fats.[205]
2. As emphasised in the American Heart Association advisory, when 'healthier' diets are incorporated in the daily routine, the amounts of saturated fat and dietary cholesterol decrease.[207]
3. If we increase nuts, fibre, green leafy vegetables, fruits, low-fat dairy and fish along with complex carbs, the amount of MUFAs and PUFAs (see Chapter 2) will increase in the diet, and the amount of cholesterol and saturated fats will decrease.
4. An additional important measure would be to decrease saturated fats as used in India (butter, dairy *ghee*, coconut oil and palm oil).

Advisory for Egg Consumption

Misra *et al.*[204] summarise thus:

1. It is reasonable to have one egg per day. The use of eggs needs to be restricted in patients with[207]:
   i. high blood cholesterol,
   ii. type 2 diabetes (poorly controlled),
   iii. heart failure and
   iv. severe heart disease of any kind.
2. There are three implications of egg consumption for India:
   i. First, for those who are vegetarian (low intake of high-quality proteins) or need more proteins to combat the low muscle mass (sarcopenia) prevalent in Indians, a higher number of eggs can be allowed. Specifically, eggs are an easily digestible source of high-quality protein, particularly leucine, which is important for skeletal

muscle synthesis. They also contain other nutrients like vitamin D and omega-3 PUFAs.

ii. Eggs could be especially beneficial for older people with sarcopenia and low nutrient intake.

iii. Early life introduction of eggs has the potential to improve growth and reduce stunting in young children, which is widely prevalent in India.

TABLE 5.9 Cholesterol Content of Dairy Products

Milk Product	Cholesterol Content (mg/100 g)
Ghee (Hybrid cow milk)	~260–275
Ghee (Sahiwal cow milk)	~260–280
Ghee (Haryana cow milk)	~270–290
Ghee (Murrah buffalo milk)	240
Cow milk (whole)	~14–16
Buffalo milk	10–12
Unsalted butter (*makhan*)	215
Processed cheese	69.3

Source: Author's own compilation.
Any differences in nutrient values reflect variations in data sources, analytical methods and preparation methods.

Summary Statement for Dietary Cholesterol Intake

1. Overall, the data generally suggests that increased dietary cholesterol influences blood cholesterol and should be particularly curbed in those with diabetes, heart failure and hypercholesterolemia.
2. Otherwise, an average intake of one egg per day is a reasonable diet choice and provides high-quality protein.
3. Healthy diet choices with plenty of MUFAs and PUFAs (see Table 2.1) and low saturated fats will help in further decreasing the intake of dietary cholesterol.
4. Dietary advice should focus on healthy dietary patterns (for example, Mediterranean-style and DASH–style diets; see Chapter 3) that are inherently relatively low in cholesterol with typical levels similar to the current US intake. These patterns emphasise fruits, vegetables, whole grains, low-fat or fat-free dairy products, lean protein sources, nuts, seeds and liquid vegetable oils.

Meats and Fishes

Meat

Meat is the flesh of animals eaten as food.

Nutrition Facts

Example: A 110 g serving of lamb contains roughly 250 Cal, 28–30 g protein, 14–20 g fat (mostly saturated) and no carbohydrates. It is also a good source of vitamin B_{12}, zinc, iron, selenium and other B vitamins, though nutrient content can vary depending on the cut and preparation (these values may vary depending on the source).

Scientific Studies

Overall, meat intake (both processed and unprocessed) is associated with an increased risk of death and multiple diseases. In general, the same may not exactly apply to non-vegetarian Indians, who generally eat less meat than the population in Western countries. Most studies focus on unprocessed red meats (beef, veal, lamb, mutton, pork and goat), which are defined as meats that are not cured, smoked or heavily processed. Despite evidence of adverse effects, recent US guidelines support meat-based diets.

Health Effects of Meat Intake

1. Cancer:
   i. Red and processed meat, but not white meat, increases the risk of gastric cancer. Higher meat consumption further increases the risk.[210]
   ii. Evidence also suggests increased risk of colorectal cancer, breast cancer and prostate cancer with red and processed meat intake.[211] [212]
2. Stroke and death: Meat intake (red meat versus white meat) increases the risk of strokes and mortality.[213]
3. Obesity: Several studies show that meat consumption is associated with increasing obesity (and associated risk factors).[214]
4. Diabetes: A robust study strongly suggests that meat consumption increases the risk of type 2 diabetes.[215]

A recent study conducted among US adults over ten years shows that reducing processed and unprocessed red meat intake could substantially lower type 2 diabetes, cardiovascular disease, colorectal (intestinal) cancer and deaths. A 30 percent reduction in both meats could prevent around 1.07 million diabetes cases, 382,000 heart disease cases, 84,000 colorectal cancer cases and 62,000 deaths. Benefits are clearer for reduction in processed meat, while effects of unprocessed red meat need further research.[216]

5. Other diseases: Some data suggests that processed meat consumption may lead to dementia.[217]
6. Some benefits:
   i. Meat eaters consume high-quality protein, which may be beneficial for Indians, who generally have weak muscles.[218]
   ii. Certain vitamins like B_{12} are sufficient in meat. Vegetarians in India generally have low levels of vitamin B_{12}.

Fish

Fish are aquatic animals eaten widely and known for several nutritional properties.

Nutrition Facts

1. Fish is an important source of protein.
2. Some fishes (labelled as 'white fish') have low fat content. Other fishes, 'oily fish' (for example, sardine, salmon and herring), contain 10–25 percent fat, and most of such fats are beneficial. These fats are mostly in the form of omega-3 PUFAs.
3. Fish also contain good amounts of vitamin D.

Omega-3 PUFAs (See Easy Reading 8 also)

Omega-3 PUFAs belong to the category of PUFAs generally considered to be fat with good effects on the body. Omega-3 PUFAs (commercially available as 'fish oil' capsules) consist of two fatty acids: eicosapentaenoic and docosahexaenoic (DHA) fatty acids. In fish oil capsules, both are mixed. These capsules are effective in lowering serum triglycerides. In addition, these oils act as anti-clotting agents and have facilitatory effects on blood flow and blood pressure (see summary of studies later). Fish oils have been tested in a variety of conditions. The benefits are the same as those listed under 'Fish'. However, the contaminants commonly associated with whole fish, including mercury, are generally not present in purified fish oil preparations. Some people do not like the smell of fish oils, and in some others, they could cause abdominal upset. Nutritional properties of fish oils are given in Table 5.10.

Scientific Studies

Many studies have been done in which generally healthy diets (for example, Mediterranean diets) include and have been supplemented with fish. Some studies (mostly from records, for example, retrospective data) have been done where fish intake has been associated with health outcomes (for example, heart disease). Other studies have evaluated the effects of purified fish oils.[219 220 221]

1. In general, the effect of omega-3 PUFAs in fish is good for the prevention of heart disease. This could be related to the amount of fish consumption. A recent major analysis (Cochrane review) also suggests that fish benefits heart disease, but more evidence is required.[220]
2. Intake of omega-3 PUFAs reduced cardiovascular mortality and improved cardiovascular outcomes. The cardiovascular risk reduction was seen with both components of omega-3 PUFAs, more so with eicosapentaenoic monotherapy.[221] However, some of these results have been contested.[222]
3. Fish oil capsules that contain omega-3 PUFAs are regularly used to decrease blood levels of triglycerides (one variety of fats in the blood).[223]
4. In a recent study, in patients with high levels of blood triglycerides (blood fats), use of ethyl ester of eicosapentaenoic (Icosapent ethyl) led to 25 percent reduction of heart disease events (see separate discussion later).[224 225]
5. It is possible that cooking methods are important. Some studies show that consumption of at least 3–4 oz servings per week of grilled or baked fish is associated with lower risk of

death by heart disease or arrhythmia, if consumed more than three times a week.[226]

6. Other effects:
   i. A few studies have suggested that fish intake or fish oil consumption is good for mental health, depression, Alzheimer's disease and so on. It has been shown to have some benefits in disorders of cognitive decline, but robust data is not available.[227]
   ii. Supplementation with omega-3 PUFAs in the third trimester of pregnancy reduced the risk of asthma and chest infections in offspring.[228]
   iii. Since these are important for nerve function and development, studies have shown short-term benefits for the brain health of children.[229]
   iv. Fish oil supplementation has been shown to increase muscle performance, mostly in women.[230]
   v. It has been shown to benefit adverse effects of pollution on the heart[231] and may have some good effects in people with skin diseases.[232]
   vi. It has been tried in joint disorders, cataract and degeneration of the macula, but results are not conclusive.
7. Some research data shows that intake of marine fish oil may increase irregularity of the heart (atrial fibrillation), but it has not been proven.

Icosapent Ethyl (A Type of Fish Oil)

Icosapent ethyl was the first fish oil product the US FDA approved to reduce the risk of atherosclerotic cardiovascular disease (heart disease) in adults. It is an esterified version of eicosapentaenoic and acts as a prodrug in the body to exert its effects. It is added to standard drugs for heart disease (statins) when triglycerides are not under control.[224 225]

TABLE 5.10 Nutritional Composition of Various Fishes Available in India

S. No	Fish/Shellfish	Hindi Name	Energy (kJ)	Protein (g)	Fat (g)	Omega-3 PUFAs (EPA) (mg)	Omega-6 PUFAs (DHA) (mg)	MUFAs (mg)
1	Catla, Carp	*Katala*	394	17.94	2.15	123	242	1,237
2	*Rohu*, Carp	*Rohu*	428	19.71	2.39	23.61	46.72	2,618
3	Silver Carp	*Sunheri rui*	555	21.71	5.17	171	125	1,964
4	Tilapia	*Tilapia*	349	18.48	1.08	14.76	59.16	254
5	Pomfret, black	*Paplet*	515	18.91	4.83	244	565	972
6	Mackerel	*Bangda*	423	21.51	1.53	72.72	259	216
7	Anchovy	*Kati*	367	19.88	0.78	60	187	50.36
8	Sardine	*Pedvey*	637	17.91	8.99	297	317	630
9	Catfish	*Singhi*	456	22.18	2.13	75.24	320	430
10	Salmon	*Rawas*	721	20.97	9.86	406	1,192	2,453
11	Tuna	*Chura*	470	24.50	1.44	90.61	345	300
12	Prawn, big	*Jhinga*	380	19.24	0.52	27.14	27.94	56.77
13	Lobster, brown	*Jhinga machhli*	292	15.96	0.56	23.17	40.06	72.73
14	Crab	*Kekda*	327	13.23	0.89	82.64	108	140

Note: All values are per 100 g portion of raw fish.
Source: Data from Longvah *et al.*[5]
Any differences in nutrient values reflect variations in data sources, analytical methods and preparation methods; EPA: Eicosapentaenoic Acid; DHA: Docosahexaenoic Acid.

Guidelines for Fish Consumption

Most dietary guidelines now include a recommendation to eat fish at least twice a week.[234]

Adverse Effects

1. Mercury content in some fishes (shark, swordfish, king mackerel or tilefish) may create potential health hazards.
2. Allergies and poisoning may occur.
3. *C. botulinum* toxin has been frequently found in canned food products.

Edible Oils

Oils are central ingredients in Indian cooking. The choice of oils and quantity of oils used daily are very important for health.

Optimal Quantity of Oils

For cooking for a single person, about 3–4 tsp per day should suffice, whichever oil is used. As opposed to carbohydrates and proteins (4 Cal/g), fats and oils contain twice the number of calories (9 Cal/g). Three tsp of oil (15 g) contain 135 Cal.

Optimal Quality of Oils

Each oil has a different quantity of types of fats.

1. The best oils are those with low saturated fatty acids, high MUFAs and high omega-3 PUFAs (see Table 5.11).
2. Consumption of just one oil is not a good idea, and a combination of oils is recommended.
3. You can choose three oils and use them in rotation, for example, each oil for ten days in a month.

Scientific Studies

1. Olive oil (*jaitoon ka tel*) has been researched most often. It is an integral part of Mediterranean diets (see Chapter 3). The following are its properties that have been scientifically investigated.[235]
    i. Olive oil is rich in monounsaturated fats, which are extremely beneficial for blood sugar, cholesterol, fat in the liver and overall heart health.

ii. Other constituents in olive oil (for example, phenolic compounds) are also important as these have antioxidant and anti-inflammatory properties.
iii. It has been hypothesised that use of this oil within healthy diets such as Mediterranean diets could delay the ageing process.[236]
iv. The evidence suggests a beneficial association between olive oil consumption and cardiovascular diseases, cancer, type 2 diabetes and all-cause mortality.[235]

2. Other oils
   i. Rice bran oil (*chawal ke chilke ka tel*) has been shown to have cholesterol-lowering properties.[237] However, a recent meta-analysis does not confirm it.[238]
   ii. Canola oil and olive oil have been shown by us to decrease liver fat and benefit metabolism.[239] [240] In addition, there was a multi-pronged effect on other associated factors such as lipids. Canola oil has also been shown to decrease abdominal fat.[241]
   iii. Mustard oil (*sarson ka tel*) is like canola oil in terms of benefits. It is low-cost and, hence, is affordable to a vast majority of the population in India. Recently, there have been some reports of gall bladder cancer with use of mustard oil.[242] A review states that cancer may occur when mustard oil is adulterated.[243] However, this needs to be confirmed.
   iv. *Desi ghee* is labelled a 'superfood', but that may not be the case.[244] Coconut oil (*nariyal ka tel*) and *desi ghee* have high saturated fat, which is deleterious to the heart and the liver. The American Heart Association has strongly recommended limiting the use of coconut oil.[222] A full discussion follows later.
   v. Similarly, palm oil (*taad ka tel*) has excess saturated fat and should be avoided. The use of palm oil has the potential to increase heart disease.[245] However, this has not been truly established.[246]
   vi. Partially hydrogenated vegetable oils (for example, *vanaspati*) contain injurious trans-fatty acids.

TABLE 5.11 Fatty Acid Composition of Commonly Available Oils in India

Fats/Oils	(% of Total Fatty Acids)			
	Saturated Fatty Acids	Monounsaturated Fatty Acids (MUFAs)	Linolenic Acid	Alpha-Linolenic Acid
Coconut oil (*nariyal ka tel*)	92	6	2	-
Palm kernel oil (*taad ke beej ka tel*)	83	15	2	-
Butter/clarified butter (*makhan*)/*ghee*	62–68	29	2	1
Olive oil (*jaitoon ka tel*)	16	71	12	1
Palm olein oil (*taad ka refine kiya hua tel*)	39	46	11	<0.5
Groundnut oil (*moongphali ka tel*)	19	41	32	<0.5
Rice bran (*chawal ke chilke ka tel*)	17	43	38	1
Sesame oil (*til ka tel*)	16	41	42	<0.5
Cottonseed oil (*kapās ke beej ka tel*)	24	29	48	1
Corn oil (*makki ka tel*)	12	35	50	1
Safflower oil (*kusum ka tel*)	9	13	75	-
Sunflower oil (*surajmukhi ka tel*)	12	22	62	-
Soybean (*soya bean ka tel*)	14	24	53	7
Canola oil	6	60	22	10
Mustard/rapeseed oil (*sarson ka tel*)	4	65	15	14
Flaxseed oil (*alsi ka tel*)	10	21	16	53
Partially hydrogenated vegetable oil★ (*vanaspati*)	46	49	4	-

Note: Content of some fatty acids in some oils may have changed since publication of the source paper mentioned here.
Source: Data from Misra *et al.*[205]
Any differences in nutrient values reflect variations in data sources, analytical methods and preparation methods.

★ Previously, *vanaspati* contained high trans fatty acids, one of the most toxic substances to health. The Food Safety and Standards Authority of India (FSSAI) capped trans-fatty acid levels in oils and fats, including *vanaspati*, at 3 percent by January 2021 and further reduced it to 2 percent or less by January 2022.[247]

Which Oils Are Suitable for Metabolism? Explanations from Table 5.11

1. High saturated fat oils such as coconut oil, palm oil, *vanaspati* (with high trans-fatty acid levels, see Table 5.11 and discussion later) and dairy *ghee* are best avoided. Use should be minimised to no more than 7 percent of total energy intake.
2. High monounsaturated fat–rich oils such as canola, olive and mustard are good for metabolism.
3. Oils with high linoleic acid (akin to omega-6 PUFAs) such as safflower, sunflower and soybean have been considered good for the heart.
4. Oils with high alpha-linolenic acid (akin to omega-3 PUFAs) are good for heart and brain health.
5. *Vanaspati* and *dalda* (partially hydrogenated vegetable oils) have high trans-fatty acid content, which is very deleterious for the heart. Recently, the government has mandated that all edible oils and fats, including *vanaspati* (partially hydrogenated vegetable oil), must contain no more than 2 percent industrially produced trans-fatty acids by weight.[247]

Coconut Oil

1. Coconut oil is widely used in South India. Many dishes are prepared with coconut/coconut oil.
2. Coconut oil contains approximately 80–90 percent saturated fatty acids, with about half of its total fat content being lauric acid (12-carbon medium-chain triglycerides; approximately 48 percent). It is believed to have high levels of medium-chain triglycerides, which is beneficial. Interestingly, excluding lauric acid, medium-chain triglycerides are around 10 percent. Lauric acid is sometimes classified as a medium-chain triglyceride, but metabolically, it behaves more like a long-chain fat, being absorbed via the lymph rather than directly through the portal vein. The remaining saturated fats include palmitic acid and other long-chain fatty acids. Coconut oil is believed to have some benefits due to MCTs, but its high saturated fat content may raise LDL cholesterol. Evidence for adverse effects, such as the promotion of cancer, is limited and not conclusive.[248 249]

3. Many people believe that coconut oil is 'good for health' (mostly because of 'high levels of medium-chain triglycerides'). It is also used in keto diets (see Chapter 3).

Scientific Studies

1. Seven controlled trials compared coconut oil with oils high in monounsaturated or polyunsaturated fats. Coconut oil raised LDL cholesterol (bad cholesterol) in all seven of these trials, significantly in six of them. It increased cholesterol more than palm oil. The authors of this study also noted that the seven trials did not find a difference in raising LDL between coconut oil and other oils high in saturated fat such as butter, beef fat or palm oil.[222 250]
2. The researchers calculated that the LDL cholesterol (a risk factor for heart disease) increase of 10.47 mg/dL from coconut oil could translate to a 6 percent increase in the risk of major vascular events (heart attack, stroke, foot gangrene) and a 5.4 percent increase in the risk of coronary heart disease mortality.[251] We also showed the overall adverse effects of coconut oil.[252]
3. Coconut oil did not significantly affect blood sugar when compared with other vegetable oils.[251]
4. One good property of coconut oil is the increase in HDL cholesterol (good cholesterol). The clinical significance of this finding is unclear.[253]
5. Interestingly, consumption of coconut flesh or squeezed coconut may not have any cardiovascular consequence.[254]
6. It has a good amount of medium-chain triglycerides, which has been showcased as the 'good' property of this oil. Medium-chain triglycerides are easily absorbable. This topic is discussed later.

Dairy Ghee

1. *Ghee* has 62 percent saturated fat (27 percent palmitic acid), 29 percent monounsaturated fat (oleic acid), about 4 percent polyunsaturated fat and 4 percent trans-fatty acids.
2. One tsp of *ghee* contains 42 Cal, 5 g fat, 0 protein, 0 carbohydrates, 0 fibre and 0 sugar. It is rich in vitamins (A, C, D, K and E).

3. *Ghee* is traditionally used in India, often daily, and frequently on special occasions. It has been referred to in Hindu mythology. In the Mahabharata, the *Kaurava*s were born from pots of *ghee*.
4. Meals made in *ghee* are usually served on special occasions. It is also believed to be good for growth (given to children and pregnant mothers), increase in strength and lubrication of joints.
5. *Ghee* is also used in *bhang* (*Cannabis sativa* leaf preparation) to heat the cannabis to cause decarboxylation.

Scientific Studies

1. Most of the studies in India and South Asia are small and not strong in design. These cannot be considered strong for any guideline for any health ailment.
2. Some studies have used the generic name *ghee* for vegetable *ghee* (*dalda*) and dairy *ghee*.
3. When examining a species of inbred rat with a genetic predisposition for various diseases, eating a *ghee*-heavy diet increased their blood's levels of unhealthy cholesterol and triglycerides.[255]
4. One human study shows that intake of dairy *ghee* (even as little as 1 tsp a day) increases the risk of heart attack several fold.[256] Another study shows it to be strongly related to occurrence of heart attacks.[257]
5. Saturated fat intake is linked to fatty liver and resultant damage; hence, *ghee* may have similar potential.[258]
6. Another recent study has shown that plasma apo B and non-HDL cholesterol (bad for the heart) are increased in those who consume *ghee* as compared with olive oil.[259]
7. Dietary guidelines for Indians clearly state to limit or avoid all saturated fats, including *ghee.*[260]
8. Clearly, it appears that *ghee* is not the superfood many people think it is. Overall, the fat properties of *ghee* are like butter. Hence, careful consumption only in small amounts is required, especially for those who have high lipids, heart disease or excess liver fat.

Medium-Chain Triglycerides

Medium-chain triglycerides are popular among nutritionists because of the purported benefits of metabolism and energy enhancement.

1. Medium-chain triglycerides (composed of six and twelve carbon molecules: C6 [caproic acid], C8 [caprylic acid], C10 [capric acid] and C12 [lauric acid]) are present in human, cow's and goat's milk as well as coconut oil and palm kernel oil. However, metabolically, lauric acid (C12) behaves more like a long-chain fatty acid than a true MCT.
2. After absorption, C6, C8 and C10 fatty acids are transported directly to the liver via the portal vein, whereas a significant portion of lauric acid (C12) is absorbed through the lymphatic system like long-chain fats. This property theoretically supports its use in malnutrition and malabsorption where people may have difficulty digesting other foods that contain long-chain triglycerides.
3. They may have beneficial anti-inflammatory, metabolic properties and weight loss properties, but the long-term effects are unknown.[261]
4. They increase the quantity of ketones in the body and, hence, may be particularly useful in supervised clinical settings such as ketogenic diets for epilepsy or metabolic disorders. Because of this property, these are part of ketogenic diets.
5. Their effect on obesity, diabetes, Alzheimer's disease[262] and epilepsy has been researched.[261]
6. They have been used for body building by sportspersons[263], although this claim has been contested.

In summary, while medium-chain triglycerides (MCTs) have been employed in weight/fat loss therapies and to enhance exercise performance, their scientific efficacy in these applications requires further investigation. Their value as a component of ketogenic diets, however, is more firmly established.[264]

Summary of Advice on Oils from Current Indian Dietary Guidelines (National Institute of Nutrition)

These guidelines advise the following:[260]

1. Use a diverse variety of oil seeds, nuts and whole grains, providing a balance of all fatty acids.
2. Minimum requirement for omega-6 PUFAs is 3 percent energy/day (6.6 g), whereas for omega-3 PUFAs, it is 0.6–1.2 percent energy/day (2.2 g).

3. Avoid intake of *ghee*/butter (*makhan*), or limit to 1–2 tsp/day. Further, it advises to include foods richer in alpha-linolenic acid/n-3 PUFAs such as nuts/dried fruits (*meve/sookhe meve*), oil seeds (*telhan beej*), soybean (*soya bean*), grains and millets (*anaj/jowar-bajra*), green leafy vegetables (*hari patte wali sabzi*) and fenugreek seeds (*methi dana*).
4. Intake of 200 g/week of marine fish such as salmon, mackerel, trout and tuna as a good source of n-3 PUFAs.
5. Minimal consumption of fast foods/ready-to-eat foods, which may contain trans-fatty acids and saturated fats.
6. Avoid using partially hydrogenated fats like *vanaspati* as a cooking medium as they contain trans-fats.
7. Avoid repeated heating of cooking oils that may generate harmful oxidative compounds.[260]

Easy Reading 13

Dietary Fats and Oils That May Make You Ill: Grandmother's Diet May Not Suit the Current Generation

Swamped with patients who have diabetes and/or are obese, it is often difficult for physicians to dispense advice on a single food item. For instance, often, we give *no* specific diktat on edible oils. This is a major gap in clinical care.

Sometimes, casual advice when patients are leaving the clinic is: 'Don't eat fried foods.' Well, that does not include putting a lot of butter on bread or plenty of *ghee* in *dal* or on *roti*s, patients gleefully think. They rationalise: How much harm can this 'little' amount do? Then they recite anecdotal evidence. 'My grandfather used to eat 100 g of *ghee* and butter daily and lived up to ninety-five years!' I explain to them that longevity is a function of a balanced lifestyle of which diet is one of the important components. 'Your grandfather must have walked 10–15 km daily and eaten plenty of vegetables, fruits and fibre-containing food. But if you are given the kind of fat he consumed, it will burst and burn your liver and heart within a short time with your current lifestyle, which is characterised by little physical activity and an uncontrolled diet.'

Both quantity and quality of the cooking oil are important. There is less controversy about the quantity of oil consumed (including cooking) daily: it should be about 3–4 tsp daily. An oil-less diet will do harm in the long run since essential fatty acids in oils are required by the body. Beware, even if a particular diet is touted to be 'zero cholesterol', there are likely to be more toxic ingredients within.

Researchers and scientists vary in their opinion about the quality of oils, but some scientific facts have emerged over the past three decades. Remarkable studies done by my colleagues from All India Institute of Medical Sciences, New Delhi, researching in the United States of America in the 1980s, showed that one component of fats, monounsaturated fat (oleic acid), when consumed instead of other fats, was highly effective in reducing blood fats and medications in patients with diabetes.[265] While this type of fat is abundant in olive (*jaitoon ka tel*) and canola oils, we have used mustard (*sarson*) oil, which is similar, for centuries. Other rich sources are avocados (*makhanphal*), pistachios (*pista*), walnuts (*akhrot*), almonds (*badam*) and sesame (*til*). The astounding success of Mediterranean diets in improving almost all health parameters, besides improving the condition of diabetics, averting heart disease and increasing lifespan, could be due to the daily use of olive oil , among other healthy food items (such as nuts, also rich in monounsaturated fats, and vegetables).

The second type of 'good' fat is polyunsaturated fat (one example is omega-3 PUFAs, found in rich levels in fish). One can face hurdles here: fish is often not available and could be contaminated (for example, with mercury). Also, many Indians do not eat fish. In general, levels of these fats are low in the blood of Indians, impacting blood fat levels and heart health adversely. Unfortunately, vegetarian sources of these good fats are few—walnuts, mustard oil, soybean, sesame, peanuts, canola oil, flaxseeds (*alsi*) and chia seeds—and contain relatively lesser amounts of omega-3 PUFAs than fish. So vegetarian people are disadvantaged.

The risk of arterial clogging and heart attacks could be extremely high due to the intake of saturated fats, though some recent opinions vary. A particularly adverse component of saturated fats is palmitic acids (high in palm oil [*taad ka tel*] and dairy *ghee*), which could also increase the growth of cancer cells (some studies are contradictory[249 266]) besides acutely increasing the risk of heart attacks. Interestingly, taking even one meal full of saturated fats could lead to an explosive break of fats deposited in arteries ('plaque rupture'), which can stop precious blood to the brain, heart or anywhere else in the body within seconds. Unfortunately, and contrary to our traditional belief ('*ghee* is good for strength and heart and lubricates joints') and our emotional attachment to it, dairy *ghee* (different from *vanaspati ghee*, which is partially hydrogenated vegetable oil made from vegetable sources, rated bad for health) and coconut oil are replete with saturated fats (60–80 percent) and palmitic acid. Hence, consuming them may do harm. Robust scientific studies on *ghee* are few, but one such study shows that a daily intake of even 1–2 tsp increases heart attack risk several fold![257] There is data to show that *ghee* increases the risk of kidney damage in animals[267] and lung cancer in human beings as well.[268] A few small studies show the good effects of *ghee* (on memory, weight and the like), but they are small and of low scientific power. Similarly, coconut oil has been found to raise bad blood cholesterol (LDL, a prime determinant of blood artery blockages) in six out of seven good studies done till date.[251] It appears that many people do not believe that coconut oil does any harm to the body, basing their opinion mostly on poorly executed small studies with little or poor scientific validity. Finally, *bhujias* (savoury fried snack) and chips widely available in India are made in palm oil, which is laden with saturated fats. Interestingly, many similar snacks (made by the same multinational companies) sold in the United States of America are made with healthier oils! All saturated fats get deposited in the liver, causing its shrinkage and damage (fibrosis and cirrhosis), something we have seen increasingly.

Surely, we all need better and more robust research data. Till then, we should decrease the intake of these oils.

Worse than saturated fats for increasing heart and liver risks are trans-fatty acids, abundant in vegetable *ghee* (*vanaspati* and many similar oils available in India). Consuming large amounts of trans-fatty acids (about 30–40 percent in some oils) is highly injurious to the heart, liver, pancreas and blood arteries. Indeed, this is the most damaging component of oil among all. Quite interestingly, our research shows that if you reheat foods at high temperatures in any oil, the levels of trans-fatty acids progressively increase by 100–200 percent. These cooking practices are common in Indian households and uniformly adopted by street vendors and most food establishments.

So how do you stay healthy? Your eyes should be open and scanning (looking at nutrition labels for quantity of saturated fats, palm oil and trans-fatty acids). You should consume more fresh fruits and vegetables and consume limited quantities of healthy oils used in rotation and in combination. You should also try not to reuse and reheat any oil.

In the polluted atmosphere that we live in, you certainly deserve one less poison.

Sugar, Sugar-Related Beverages and Artificial Sweeteners

Sugar

Sugar is believed to have been invented in India. Sweets are a customary way to celebrate any joyous occasion. Nutritionally, sugar provides only 'empty' calories (1 g of sugar gives 4 Cal). See Table 5.12 for subgroups and components of sugar.

TABLE 5.12 Types of Dietary Sugars

Sugars: Subgroups	Principal Components
Monosaccharides	Glucose, fructose, galactose
Disaccharides	Sucrose (glucose and fructose), lactose (glucose and galactose), maltose (glucose and glucose), trehalose (glucose and glucose)
Free sugars	All monosaccharides and disaccharides added to foods by the manufacturer, cook or consumer; sugars naturally present in honey, syrups and fruit juices

Source: Data from Gulati and Misra.[269]

Sugar-sweetened beverages (SSBs, *shakkar yukt pey*) include the full spectrum of aerated drinks, fruit drinks and energy and vitamin water drinks containing added sugars. Some of these are sweetened by HFCS.

There are several traditional sugars in India, produced from sugarcane. Jaggery (*gur*) is obtained by boiling clarified sugarcane juice till a solid residue is left after evaporation. It usually contains 65–85 percent sucrose and is also a source of calcium, potassium and iron. *Khandsari* is a finely granulated crystallised sugar that contains 94–98 percent sucrose. It is less refined than sugar and retains some calcium.

In general, excess intake of sugar is considered bad for health. Currently, it is recommended to consume sugar less than 10 percent of the total food being consumed per day. Ideally, sugar should be consumed in quantities less than 5 percent of the total energy intake per day or 25 g per day (based on average intake of 2,000 Cal/day).[260]

Ultra-processed foods are often high in fat, sugar and salt. Overall, compared with people with low consumption of ultra-processed food, those with the highest consumption have been shown to have higher risks of type 2 diabetes, hypertension, overweight or obesity, cardiovascular (heart attacks) and cerebrovascular events (stroke) as well as all-cause and cardiovascular mortality (deaths due to any cause and heart disease).[270]

TABLE 5.13 Commonly Consumed Sugar-Containing Food Articles in India

Main Meals	Snacks	Beverages	Add-On
All carbohydrates: rice, wheat (*gehu*), buckwheat (*kuttu*), oats (*jai*), millets, barley (*jau*), breads, sugar/jaggery (*gur*)-stuffed Indian bread, yoghurt (*dahi*) and vegetables	Indian sweets (*halwa, kheer* and so on), *kulfi* (frozen milk dessert), *chikki* (peanut candy), puddings, fruit cakes, biscuits, ice creams and processed foods	Sugarcane juice, *shikanji* (Indian spiced lemon-ade), sweetened buttermilk (*chaach*), *sharbat* (syrup drink), *aam panna* (raw mango drink), milkshakes, fruit juices, SSBs and so on	Sweet *chutneys* (dip or sauce), pickles (*achaar*), *aamras* (mango pulp), *murabbas* (sweet preserve), honey, *khandsari* (unre-fined cane sugar) with *ghee,* jams, tomato (*tamatar*) ketchup and so on

Source: Data from Gulati and Misra.[269]
Note: SSBs refer to sugar-sweetened beverages.

Sugar-Sweetened Beverages (SSBs)

SSBs are beverages with added sugar.

Health Concerns and Scientific Studies

1. Since most SSBs have added sugar, concerns for weight gain, development of diabetes, liver disease (non-alcoholic fatty liver disease or MASLD, indicating excess toxic fat accumulation in liver), type 2 diabetes and heart disease have been shown in various studies. Indeed, many studies show SSBs increased the risk of diabetes and heart disease independent of weight gain.[271 272]
2. Fruit drinks with added sugar and even 100 percent fruit juices (due to high free sugar and low fibre) may have adverse metabolic effects when consumed in excess.
3. Even if low-calorie sweeteners (non-nutritive sweeteners [NNS]) are added to beverages to reduce concerns about weight gain, NNSs may promote appetite and cause weight gain. This decision is still controversial and needs extensive research with a special focus on alteration of the gut microbiome, which is responsible for glucose metabolism and satiety factors of food.
4. SSBs have been linked to tooth decay.

5. Rarely, the excessive intake of cola-type beverages has also been linked to low potassium levels.

Fruit Juices

1. In general, sugar-sweetened fruit juices are not recommended as a part of a healthy diet; instead, whole fruits are better.
2. A small quantity of fresh juices (preferably a mixture of fruits and vegetables) as a part of a healthy diet may decrease heart-related risk factors.
3. Benefits of some fruit juices:
   i. In some studies, beetroot juice (*chukandar ka ras*) lowered blood pressure. Nitrate supplementation from this may also increase endurance during exercise and decrease fatigue.[273]
   ii. Cranberry juice intake may help in preventing/decreasing urinary tract infections, especially in women.[274]
   iii. Pomegranate (*anar*) polyphenols, when present in a beverage but not in a supplement, can reduce the postprandial blood sugar when taken with foods with high glycaemic index values.[275]
   iv. Tomato (*tamatar*) juice has been shown to increase antioxidant levels.[276]

Artificial Sweeteners

Artificial sweeteners (*kritrim mithaas*), also known as sugar substitutes or NNSs, are chemicals or food additives that duplicate the effect of sugar in taste but contain fewer calories/less energy. Artificial sweeteners available in India (approved by the US FDA) are as follows:

1. Sucralose: It is also marketed under the name Splenda (available as powder and pellets).
2. Aspartame: It is also sold under the brands Equal (Equal may not always contain aspartame) and NutraSweet (available as powder and pellets).
3. Saccharin: It is also known as Sweet'N Low (available as powder, pellets and liquid).
4. Acesulfame Potassium: It is also known as acesulfame-K, Ace-K or Sweet One (available as powder).
5. Neotame: It is like aspartame. It is not available under any brand yet.

6. Advantame: It was approved in 2014 by FDA. It is a high-intensity sweetener derived from aspartame and vanillin. It is primarily used in food manufacturing instead of being commonly sold as a tabletop sweetener.
7. Stevia: It is sold with many brand names and is available as powder and liquid extraction. The sweetening agents are purified steviol glycosides derived from the stevia plant. These plant-derived non-nutritive sweeteners are considered generally safe within recommended intake limits, although long-term metabolic effects are still being studied.
8. Others such as sugar alcohols (for example, sorbitol, erythritol), monk fruit extract and lucuma powder are also available. Sugar alcohols, when consumed in excess, can cause gastrointestinal discomfort, while monk fruit extract is a high-intensity natural sweetener with limited long-term data.

Generally Safe Intake

A safe quantity of artificial sweeteners is 2–3 pellets, 2–3 g powder (½ tsp), 2–3 sachets or 5 drops of liquid. If possible, avoid these sweeteners.

Adverse Effects

Overuse of artificial sweeteners can cause health problems, though none of them are common:

1. Laxative effect, bloating of abdomen
2. Weight gain (rare)
3. Increase in bone loss
4. Increase in blood glucose levels, heart disease and cancer susceptibility (recently believed but not confirmed; see Easy Reading 13 below)

Other General Points for Sweets and Artificial Sweeteners

1. Limit the intake of sugar-free foods (like chocolate, diet coke, baked goods) as they contain sugar alcohols, fructose, saccharin and maltodextrin, which are not sugar but are high in carbohydrates, which affect blood glucose levels.
2. Children and those who are pregnant or lactating should avoid using artificial sweeteners. Children with phenylketonuria should never consume artificial sweeteners.

3. Recent data, however, shows that the use of artificial sweeteners by non-diabetic individuals does not help in weight loss and may increase the risk of metabolic diseases, including diabetes.[277 278] However, as listed, only limited quantities of these sweeteners should be used till more research is available.

Easy Reading 14

Artificial Sweeteners: More Bitter than Sweet for Health?

'I always drink diet colas and take two helpings of artificial sweeteners for the seven to eight cups of tea and coffee that I drink daily, Doc, yet I am gaining weight.' Tread carefully here, I advise a thirty-year-old female patient.

Many of us have a sweet tooth and look for a replacement for sugar. Artificial sweeteners look like the simple answer, but there are more problems than meet the tongue here. Research has revealed some troublesome problems.

Artificial sweeteners, also called non-nutritive sweeteners (NNS, because these have no nutrition potential), are mostly chemically made. They are 30–1,300 times sweeter than natural sugar, sucrose. These are used in the preparation of sweetened beverages, juices, dairy products, desserts, processed foods, jams and so on. There are several artificial sweeteners: aspartame, saccharin, sucralose, neotame, cyclamate, acesulfame-K, stevia, erythritol and so on. The first five of these have been generally recognised as safe (GRAS) by the FDA, United States of America. Stevia, a plant-based sweetener, has been used in Japan since the 1970s but has not yet been approved by the FDA. These artificial sweeteners have been promoted as diabetes- and tooth-friendly and for inducing weight loss.

Development of Artificial Sweeteners Was Beset with Problems

The story of saccharin is widely known. It was used in both World Wars for sugar rationing. In laboratory animals, it was found to induce bladder cancer. This doubt was later cleared with further studies. Aspartame is toxic to patients who suffer from a rare disorder, phenylketonuria. It has been blamed for brain tumours, chronic fatigue syndrome and so on without any concrete proof. The fear of cancer with the use of saccharin still lingered in people's minds.

Uncertainty Continues: Artificial Sweeteners May Not Be Beneficial for Weight or Diabetes

All individuals using artificial sweeteners aim to cut down calories by doing so. Thus, they expect weight loss and anticipate decrease, or at least no increase, in blood sugar. They believe it will lead to a general improvement in health due to the absence of sugar in the diet. However, some studies now show that use of these agents leads to obesity, hypertension, type 2 diabetes and even strokes upon long-term use, contrary to expectations. However, others continue to vouch for their effectiveness. In a recent review, authors of a major study state: 'The available evidence suggests that NNS beverages sweetened with single or blends of NNS have no acute metabolic and endocrine effects, similar to water', thus supporting the use of these agents in beverages.[279]

However, the authors of a major review published in 2019 cautioned that the quality of most studies on artificial sweeteners was not of a high standard. After considering data from all studies, they concluded that 'no evidence was seen for health benefits from non-sugar sweeteners and potential harms could not be excluded'.[280] A World Health Organization (WHO) review (2022) also concluded that long-term weight loss has not been proven with the use of artificial sweeteners. Beverages/cola companies have opposed this notion.[277]

The following studies raise fresh concerns.

New Signals of Cancer and Heart Disease with Intake of Artificial Sweeteners

In a recent large French study (NutriNet-Santé, published in 2022), people taking artificial sweeteners were studied for nearly eight years. In this study, the overall risk of cancers (breast cancer and obesity-associated cancers) was shown to be increased, correlating to the amount of intake of these sweeteners.[281] This result was particularly shown for aspartame and acesulfame-K, which have been used in a wide variety of popular foods and beverages worldwide. In this study, most people consumed sweetened beverages or tabletop sweeteners. An interesting point is whether weight gain associated with artificial sweeteners leads to an observed increase in cancer risk. Possible cellular mechanisms for induction of cancer include inflammation and DNA damage.

A more damaging recent study (published in a top journal, *Nature Medicine*) shows that the artificial sweetener erythritol (sold singly or combined with other artificial sweeteners such as stevia) can induce thrombosis (clotting), thus having the potential to cause heart attacks or strokes over three years. More concerning, once taken, erythritol can stay in the body for several days. This study was very well conducted and consists of population-based and lab-based data.[282] Increase in heart disease and stroke risk due to artificial sweeteners (aspartame, acesulfame, sucralose) has been shown by a large (103,388 participants) French study published in 2022.[283] Concerned by the findings of these recent studies, many people suggest that FDA and other regulatory agencies should revise their guidelines as to which artificial sweeteners should be considered generally safe/unsafe. A recent WHO guideline summarised all evidence to state that these artificial sweeteners should not be used for weight control or for reducing risk for non-communicable diseases such as diabetes.[277]

My Advisory about Artificial Sweeteners Has Changed

In view of recent data, I often worry about uninformed individuals who continue to take sweetened beverages in excess. I also wonder if some of these artificial sweeteners are being mixed in *laddoo*s and *mithai*s (sweets) targeted at people with diabetes during festivals, especially Diwali. I am also worried if these artificial sweeteners have been put in particularly sweet fruits I recently bought.

However, I am clearer in my mind as to my advice. I agree with the French researchers of two large studies[283 284]: 'Our results indicate that these food additives, consumed daily by millions of people and present in thousands of foods and beverages, should not be considered a healthy and safe alternative to sugar.'[285]

No artificial sweeteners from now on and that includes diet colas, I tell my patients. I allow patients with well-controlled diabetes to take less than 5 g sugar (about 1 tsp) in tea/coffee instead. Finally, I have made a mental note to carefully read the package labels of all sweet foods I buy, including those of chocolates, a luxury I sometimes indulge in.

Note: This article, originally featured in *The Indian Express*, has been revised and updated from its initial published version.

Honey

Honey (*shahad*) is a sweet and viscous liquid made by honeybees from plants. It has fructose (about 38 percent), glucose (31 percent) and several other sugars. It is as sweet as table sugar (sucrose).

Popular Health-Centric Uses

1. Honey has been traditionally used to treat wounds because of its 'antibacterial property'. It has been used in patients with diabetes who have wounds on their feet.
2. Some effect has been demonstrated in burns as well.
3. It may be a beneficial therapy for cough.

Adverse Properties

1. Although it has lower GI than glucose, it may increase blood sugars in patients with diabetes.[286] There are some studies that indicate that it may stimulate insulin secretion.[287] Honey had less effect on serum glucose than the honey-comparable glucose-fructose solution.[288] Due to the lack of good-quality studies, firm conclusions cannot be drawn. Patients with diabetes may take small amounts of honey, but large quantities must be avoided.
2. There is a danger of botulism (a dangerous disease) in contaminated (with bacteria *C. botulinum*) honey.

High-Fructose Corn Syrup (HFCS)

HFCS is a commonly used sweetener (alternative to sugar) industrially produced by processing starch from corn. It has about 76 percent carbohydrates, about 24 percent water, and no other nutrients. Commercial forms include HFCS-42 (about 42 percent fructose) and HFCS-55 (about 55 percent fructose), with the remainder primarily glucose. Its sweetness is similar to that of sucrose, and it is stable and easy to use in processed foods.

HFCS is widely used in soft drinks (typically with HFCS-55 as the sweetener), breakfast cereals, pancake syrup, canned fruits, flavored yogurts, jams and jellies.

Health Implications

1. Several recent studies show that blood glucose excursions after HFCS are like fructose or honey. A study in Taiwan found that it has high GI (73 percent of glucose).[289] It may increase hunger and overeating.
2. A meta-analysis considered that ingestion of HFCS is related to adverse effects on fatty liver (which may be related to concurrent excess calorie intake), but evidence was not robust.[290]
3. It may increase the risk for heart disease.[291]
4. Overall, HFCS seems to be metabolically unfavourable, but more data is needed.

Healthy Snacks

1. In India, there is a general habit of snacking, sometimes excessively, in between meals. Fried snacks are often preferred. There are occasions where such snacks are preferentially prepared: monsoon season, parties, weddings, meetings and when drinking alcohol.
2. Limited calories must be consumed from snacks to avoid weight gain and destabilisation of diabetes.
3. In general, the calorie value of snacks should be below 100 Cal to keep hunger pangs at bay and the energy levels high. Here are some basic principles:
   i. Apple (*seb*), pear (*nashpati*) and low-fat fruit yoghurt are good snacks.
   ii. Go for roasted and baked *namkeens* (salty snacks), five to eight almonds (*badam*), pistachios (*pista*) or one to two walnuts, a handful of puffed rice or eight to ten roasted peanuts (*moongphali*).

iii. A protein shake/drink could decrease appetite and boost metabolism if kidney function is normal.
iv. Avoid biscuits and cookies as they contain a considerable amount of shortening, salt and sugar.

4. Table 5.14 gives a list of healthy snacks that are also suitable for patients with diabetes or high cholesterol values.

TABLE 5.14 Nutritive Value of Some Commonly Consumed Snacks

Healthy Snacks	Energy (Cal)	Protein (g)	Carbohy-drate (g)	Fibre (g)
Buttermilk (*chaach*) (200 ml = 1 glass)	30	1.6	1	0
Tender coconut water (*nariyal paani*)	41	0.9	6.3	0
Fruit (strawberry/*stroberee*) 100 g	44	0.7	9.8	2
Walnuts (*akhrot*) (8 g = 5 halves)	55	1.2	0.9	0.5
Flaxseeds (*alsi*) (1 tbsp)	55	3.1	4	3.8
Pistachios (*pista*) (15 pcs)	58	2.2	2.9	1.1
Protein biscuits (15 g = 3 biscuits)	63.3	13.5	7.2	0.6
Almonds (*badam*) (12 g = 12 pcs)	80	2.5	6.6	1.4
Protein cookies (20 g = 2 cookies)	93	1.9	11.7	1
Flattened rice with vegetables (*poha*) (100 g = 1 *katori* cooked)	96.5	6.8	23	3
Roasted chickpeas (*bhuna chana*) (1 handful)	101	7	17	3.3

Source: Author's own compilation.
Any differences in nutrient values reflect variations in data sources, analytical methods and preparation methods.

Miscellaneous Food Items

Popcorn

Popcorn is made by heating corn kernels, which then puff up. Various forms of popcorns are available with different artificial flavours or added butter. It is usually consumed as a leisure snack while watching movies. Most of the popcorn available in movie halls contains a good amount of butter or other calorie-rich additives.

Nutrition Facts

1. A serving of 100 g air-popped popcorn contains 382 Cal energy, 78 g carbohydrates (15 g fibre), 4 g fat and 12 g protein.
2. Three cups (small bowl) of air-popped popcorn contain 93 Cal; when buttered, the same quantity contains 192 Cal.
3. A large popcorn (movie theatre size) is equal to sixteen to twenty cups of popcorn, 1,000–1,200 Cal and about 60 g of saturated fats. Many theaters pop their corn in coconut oil, which is extremely high in saturated fat, and 60g is roughly three days' worth of the recommended daily limit for saturated fat.

Health Implications

There are no proper scientific trials on popcorn and health. However, the consumption of a small quantity of popcorn may have some metabolic benefit due to the high amount of fibre and protein.

Green Tea

Green tea (*hari chai*) is made from *Camellia sinensis* leaves and buds. This kind of tea is not subjected to withering and oxidation processes as is done for oolong teas (from China) and black teas.

Nutrition Facts

1. A 100 g serving of unsweetened brewed tea contains approximately 1 Cal, 0.32 g carbohydrates, 0.01 g protein and 0 g fat. The nutritional content is minimal and can vary slightly depending on the tea type and brewing method.
2. It is rich in polyphenols and catechin. Catechins are the major polyphenolic compounds in green tea, which include epigallocatechin-3-gallate (EGCG), epigallocatechin, epicatechin-3-gallate and epicatechin, gallocatechins and gallocatechin gallate. EGCG is the predominant and most studied catechin in green tea.

3. Polyphenols, particularly catechins, are powerful antioxidants that may help protect the body against damage from free radicals (harmful unstable molecules), potentially reducing the risk of chronic diseases.

Scientific Studies

In general, green tea consumption is believed to be healthy and safe.

1. Claims have been made about the effects of green tea on cancer, heart disease, diabetes, hypertension and mortality in kidney disease,[292 293] but results have been inconsistent. Potential benefits appear with higher-than-usual consumption, typically more than two to three cups per day.[294]
2. There is some evidence to suggest that green tea causes marginal reduction in lipid levels. The total cholesterol is reduced by 2 percent and LDL cholesterol by 4 percent. Reviews and trials state that it reduces lipids and blood sugar, but more studies are needed.[295 296]
3. Green tea is popularly taken for weight loss. In some studies, it has been shown to promote weight loss, but the extent of weight loss is minimal at best. Similar conclusions were reached in 2012 in a Cochrane review.[297]
4. There is some evidence to suggest that green tea intake helps in reducing the risk for dementia and Alzheimer's disease and improves memory.[298]
5. Green tea may activate brown fat, which stimulates metabolism in the body.[299]
6. It has been shown to reduce knee pain and increase mobility in osteoarthritis (age-related arthritis) of the knee.[300]
7. An interesting study proposes that gargling with green tea may decrease influenza.[301]
8. Another study shows that daily consumption leads to increase in the muscles' aerobic capacity, that is, functioning of muscles.[302]
9. Studies have shown possible effects on breast, prostate, colorectal, skin and lung cancers.[294]

Black Tea

Black tea is also known to improve post-meal sugar status.[303]

Caution

Very hot tea has been shown to increase the risk of oesophageal and gastric cancers.

Chocolates

Chocolates are made from dried/roasted cocoa seeds. Their consumption was considered to be bad for health, thought to be associated with acne, caries, obesity, high blood pressure, coronary artery disease and diabetes.[304] Most dark chocolate is rich in flavanols (antioxidants) that may confer health benefits.

The following are three common varieties:

1. Milk: contains ~20 percent cocoa
2. White: does not contain non-fat cocoa
3. Dark: cocoa content about 35 percent

Nutrition Facts

1. Per 100 g, chocolate provides approximately 540 Cal, 59 g carbohydrates (including 51 g sugars and 3–7 g fibre), 7–8 g protein and 30 g fat. It contains useful amounts of magnesium, manganese, iron and B vitamins. Caffeine content varies (around 20 mg in milk chocolate, higher in dark varieties). Sugar content varies by type (higher in milk chocolate, lower in dark chocolate). Cholesterol is present only in milk chocolate (around 20 mg/100 g) but not in pure dark chocolate (these values may vary depending on the source).
2. It contains biologically active phenolic compounds, especially epicatechin. Because of the bitter taste, manufacturers use processing techniques that may eliminate up to 90 percent of the flavonoids.

Scientific Studies

Possible Benefits

1. Flavanol in chocolates may decrease cell damage.[305]
2. Some studies show that flavanol ingestion may cause lowering of blood pressure and elasticity of arteries and benefit the heart,[306] [307] but these effects not been conclusively proven.[308]

3. There is no effect on the brain and the psychological system due to short-term chocolate consumption.
4. In a recent major review, calorie-balanced greater consumption of chocolate was inversely associated with lower heart disease and cancer mortality (deaths).[309] These findings need further investigation.
5. Effects of dark chocolates have often been floated in the media, but many of them are exaggerated. Dark chocolate is distinguished from milk chocolate by its higher concentration of cocoa solids (typically 70 percent or higher) and the absence of milk solids. While still calorie-dense, it is globally recognised as a functional food due to its rich profile of bioactive compounds. The following are statements from some scientific studies:
   i. Cholesterol, triglycerides and abdominal obesity were improved after six months of daily intake of 2 g of dark chocolate with 70 percent cocoa as compared to milk chocolates.[305]
   ii. Dark chocolates, and not milk chocolates, decrease the risk of type 2 diabetes.[310]
   iii. It may benefit fatty liver.[311]
   iv. There is some evidence that ingestion of dark chocolates may acutely decrease appetite[312] likely due to the presence of epicatechin.
   v. It has been shown to have anti-inflammatory effects.[313]

Bad Effects on Health due to Chronic Excess Consumption of Chocolates

1. Chocolate ingestion has been linked to acne, dental caries, heartburn and kidney stones.
2. Because of caffeine content, pulse rate may go up. There is also a remote possibility of destabilisation of heart rhythm (cardiac arrhythmia). However, some research shows that a particular type of heart irregularity (atrial fibrillation) may decrease with moderate chocolate consumption.[314]
3. Chocolate is generally not advised in diabetic patients; if taken, only small portions of high-cocoa dark chocolate may be allowed occasionally.

Ginkgo Biloba

Ginkgo biloba is a tree traditionally used for both medicinal purposes and food. The edible nut, found inside the tree's seeds, is commonly consumed in various countries, particularly in China and Japan.

Nutrition Facts

Ginkgo biloba is rich in flavonoids and terpenoids, which accounts for its antioxidant capacity.

Popular Health-Centric Uses

1. Ginkgo biloba is used as a health supplement, specially to increase memory and 'brain power'.
2. It has also been used for fighting infections and improving sexual energy.

Scientific Studies

1. Ginkgo biloba has been used extensively in brain disorders, including Alzheimer's disease. A review suggests that it may have some role in the treatment of mild cognitive disorders only if given for more than twenty-four weeks and at a defined dose,[315] but results of other studies are conflicting.
2. It may have some effects on depression.[316]
3. There are a few studies that indicate that it may have some effects on tinnitus ('ringing in the ear'), but this has not been proven.[317]

Caution

1. Consumption of ginkgo biloba may increase chances of bleeding because of its effects on coagulation. So it must be taken with caution or avoided in patients on aspirin or other anticoagulants (patients with heart disease or diabetes).[318]
2. In animal studies, there is some signal for increased cancer risk with this compound.[319]

Apple Cider Vinegar

Apple cider vinegar is vinegar made from the juice of crushed apples (*seb*).

Nutrition Facts

Per 100 g, apple cider vinegar contains 22 Cal, 0.93 g carbohydrates (0.4 g sugar, 0 g fibre), 0 g protein and 0 g fat. It is devoid of any vitamins.

Scientific Studies

Some studies have been done with vinegar, which are also summarised. It is popular in people aiming for weight loss.

1. It has been shown to have antimicrobial properties.[320]
2. Although it is popularly believed to aid weight loss, this effect has not been conclusively demonstrated, and surprisingly few studies have investigated it. Some studies have shown the beneficial properties of vinegar on blood sugar, especially on post-meal spikes.[321 322 323 324]
3. One systematic review found that patients with type 2 diabetes who took apple cider vinegar less than 15ml/day for more than eight weeks had a significant reduction in total cholesterol levels, triglyceride levels and fasting blood glucose. It also showed an increase in HDL (good cholesterol) levels in healthy people.[324]

Caution

1. The acid content of apple cider vinegar may vary in products, and excess acid has the potential to cause tongue, throat and oesophagus injury.[325]
2. Anecdotal reports suggest that if the person is taking insulin or diuretics, having apple cider vinegar can lead to low potassium levels.[326]
3. In patients with type 1 diabetes, it may cause the bowels to become sluggish.[327]

Ginseng

Ginseng is the root of a plant found in eastern Asia.

Popular Health-Centric Uses

In Korea, China and other Asian countries, ginseng has been traditionally used as a medicine. It is used in soups, beverages and liquor. It is taken for strength and vitality, especially in men over fifty years of age in China.

Scientific Studies

There are a number of studies, mostly from East Asia, about the effects of ginseng on cancer, heart disease, blood pressure and so on. The results are inconclusive.

1. There is some data that ginseng could reduce fatigue based on an analysis of several studies,[328] although this statement has been disputed by others.
2. It has no effect on the treatment of respiratory disorders like chronic obstructive pulmonary disease (damaged lung),[329] although previously some effects were observed on common cold.[330]
3. Although some studies have shown ginseng's beneficial properties for blood glucose and insulin, others have not shown any benefit.[331]
4. In women, some effects on post-menopausal symptoms have been shown.[332]
5. It has been said to have beneficial effects on quality of life and psychological well-being in healthy young adults, but this statement has not been generally supported by many studies.[333]
6. It has been shown to improve sexual health, mostly in women,[334] but this needs to be tested in more studies.

Caution

1. Many commercial products of ginseng may have contaminants harmful to the body.[335]
2. In some people, it may cause nervousness, insomnia, changes in blood pressure, vomiting and diarrhoea.[335]

Easy Reading 15

Processed and Ultra-Processed Foods: Unseen Poisons

'Doc, when I travel abroad, I take a lot of pre-packaged Indian food with me. Is that good?' 'My son eats packaged noodles for each meal. Will it harm his growth and health?' Such questions to me are increasing daily, and so is the consumption of processed foods. In India, consumption of processed foods has doubled since 2012.

What Are Processed and Ultra-Processed Foods?

Any food that is altered in some physical or chemical way (mostly industrial) is termed as processed food (*prasanskrut khadya padarth*). When five or more industrial formulations are added using sophisticated industrial equipment, it is called ultra-processed food. After cleaning, freezing, parboiling and frying, several ingredients are added, which is the most harmful step for health. Some of these ingredients include whey protein, gluten, casein, lactose, hydrogenated oils, hydrolysed proteins, soy protein isolate, maltodextrin, invert sugar and high-fructose corn syrup. Then these foods, in attractive packages, are ready for all convenience stores and super bazaars. The processing of various foods increases their taste and shelf life.

Common examples of processed foods include canned vegetables, frozen fruits, plain yogurt, cheese and freshly baked bread, and ultra-processed foods include breakfast cereals, canned products, instant soups, instant meals/noodles, flavoured potato chips, flavoured candy bars, energy bars, table sauces, reconstituted meats (for example, sausages) and so on. Some examples of ultra-processed foods available and consumed in India include packaged baby cereals, packaged fruit juices and sweetened carbonated beverages, energy drinks, sweet Indian packaged snacks, 'health' drinks, most biscuits and prepared pastas or pizzas. The only 'good' part is that these foods taste good, and many people are addicted to them.

What Are the Harmful Ingredients in Processed Foods?

There could be multiple problems with consumption of processed foods. These are high in calories, salt and sugar. More importantly, these foods are high in trans-fats, a form of fat that is highly damaging to human health. Good nutrients such as protein and fibre are generally low.

Additionally, these foods contain harmful additives and newly formed compounds. Further, the packaging may contain chemicals known as hormone disruptors, which may affect health in a yet unknown manner. For example, the following elements could be damaging to health:

1. Carrageenan and carboxymethylcellulose are thickening agents commonly employed in meat and dairy product formulations, which have been shown to be associated with intestinal inflammation.
2. Emulsifiers and stabilisers are commonly added to processed foods and have the potential to cause metabolic disturbances.
3. Packaging contaminants include synthetic compounds like bisphenol A, which is widely present in food packaging, and phthalates, which are another class of synthetic chemicals commonly used in food packaging. Bisphenol A has the potential to impair reproductive function in men and increase cancer risk, while phthalates have the potential to act as xenohormones (chemicals which could produce human hormone-like effects).

What Are the Bad Health Outcomes of Processed Foods?

One outcome that is consistent across many studies is weight gain. This is mostly seen in young individuals and is particularly worrisome for India, where childhood obesity is on the rise. A closely related association is metabolic syndrome, a conglomeration of various risk factors including obesity (specifically excess abdominal fat), high blood pressure, high blood sugar and deranged cholesterol profile. Currently, about one-third of the urban Indian population has this syndrome. This metabolic syndrome is a forerunner to heart disease. A few studies show that excessive consumption of processed foods is linked to bowel irregularity. While COVID-19 has increased the number of people with mental health problems, depression has also been linked to processed foods.

However, there are more severe outcomes linked to processed foods: diabetes is one, and heart disease, stroke and deaths due to any cause are the other dangerous ones. Further research is just beginning on many other outcomes like cancers.

I Fear Eating Processed Foods. What Do I Eat Now?

Many patients ask me, 'Doc, eating is one of the prime pleasures of life. How can I stop eating my food like this?'

My usual answer is, 'Limit your processed food intake to one day a week, and the rest of the days, eat more unprocessed foods. Read the labels while buying any packaged foods from the market, thus limiting your choices to those with least salt, sugar and fat contents.' I further emphasise that the industry advertising (often by celebrities) is mostly misleading and not to go by them. Genuine sources of information include the WHO, Government of India and some public interest groups.

Finally, and most importantly, have 'real food'. These include unprocessed foods such as fresh fruits, vegetables, whole grains, nuts, meat, legumes, curds (*dahi*) (not flavoured yoghurt) and milk. Cook at home the traditional way but with healthy oils with less saturated fats, and eat fresh.

Note: This article, originally featured in *The Indian Express*, has been revised and updated from its initial published version.

List of Processed and Ultra-Processed Foods

Processed foods are those that have been altered from their natural state for convenience, safety or shelf stability. This can include a wide range of items, from minimally processed to heavily processed. Here are some common categories and examples of processed foods.

Minimally Processed Foods

These foods are often processed for preservation or convenience but retain most of their nutritional value.

1. Washed and packaged fruits and vegetables (for example, pre-cut salad greens, baby carrots [*gajar*])
2. Roasted nuts and seeds
3. Canned beans (without added sugar or salt)
4. Frozen fruits and vegetables (without added ingredients)

Foods Processed for Preservation or Safety

These foods have undergone processes like canning, freezing or drying to extend their shelf life.

1. Canned vegetables and fruits

2. Frozen meals and entrées
3. Dried fruits
4. Canned fish (for example, tuna, salmon)

Foods with Added Ingredients

These foods have added ingredients such as sweeteners, oils, colours and preservatives to enhance flavour, texture or shelf life.

1. Breakfast cereals, cornflakes, muesli
2. Packaged bread and baked goods
3. Instant noodles
4. Canned soups

Heavily (Ultra) Processed Foods

These foods are often far removed from their natural state and may contain many added ingredients and artificial substances.

1. Snack foods (for example, chips, pretzels, cheese puffs)
2. Sugary drinks (for example, sodas, energy drinks)
3. Processed meats (for example, sausages, hot dogs, deli meats)
4. Ready-to-eat meals (for example, frozen dinners, microwaveable ready-to-eat meals)

Sweets and Desserts

These foods are typically high in sugar and fat and are usually ultra-processed.

1. Candy
2. Ice cream
3. Cookies and cakes
4. Pastries

Condiments and Sauces

These are often processed or ultra-processed, used to enhance flavour and extend shelf life, and may contain added sugar, salt, unhealthy fats, preservatives or flavour enhancers.

1. Ketchup
2. Mayonnaise
3. Salad dressings
4. Soy sauce

Beverages

Processed beverages can range from minimally processed to ultra-processed, depending on the ingredients and the manufacturing method.

1. Juices (especially those with added sugars and flavours)
2. Sports drinks
3. Flavoured milk and milk alternatives

Instant and Convenience Foods

These foods are designed for quick and convenient preparation, and are often classified as processed or ultra-processed, depending on the added ingredients.

1. Instant coffee
2. Instant oatmeal
3. Microwave popcorn
4. Pre-packaged sandwiches

This list includes a wide spectrum of processed foods, varying in the degree of processing and the presence of added ingredients. While some processed foods can be part of a healthy diet, others, especially those high in added sugars, salts and fats, should be consumed in moderation.

6

Supplements and Vitamins

Dietary Supplements

1. Dietary supplements are meant to supplement nutrients to diets. In recent times, the sales of dietary supplements have increased substantially.
2. The constituents of dietary supplements include minerals, vitamins, fibre, botanicals, herbs, oils, enzymes and similar substances.
3. In India, many supplements contain elements from alternative systems of medicine (for example, Ayurveda).
4. Many vitamin supplements contain a mixture of vitamins, minerals and other elements, sometimes thirty or more. Most of these are not needed by the body.
5. Many such supplements are not quality-controlled, that is, do not undergo rigorous testing to detect the exact dose or impurities.
6. Hence, many impurities are detected in such supplements, sometimes inadvertent and often deliberate (for example, mixing of steroids or sex hormones).

Should I Take Dietary Supplements/Vitamins? (See also Easy Reading 1)

1. It depends on age, existing diseases, dietary patterns and the presence of deficiencies.
2. An individual who is free of any disease and is eating largely healthy diets with plenty of fruits and vegetables and balanced portions of proteins, dairy and a variety of other foods does not need any extra supplements. Supplements can never replace healthy diets.

3. However, in the following situations, supplements may be needed.
   i. Older and frail individuals may need more proteins, calcium and vitamins.
   ii. For people having low appetite, vomiting or diarrhoea, almost all nutrients are needed. Sometimes these are given by intravenous lines or nasogastric tube (feeding tube through the nose).
   iii. People suffering from cancer, kidney disease and liver disease need multiple nutrients.
   iv. Pregnant women require multiple nutrients, importantly, folic acid.
   v. People having malabsorption (poor absorption of nutrients from the intestine), of nutrients, intestinal disease and pancreatitis (inflammation of the pancreas) need multiple supplements.
   vi. People having prolonged fever, tuberculosis or similar chronic diseases need protein and vitamins.
   vii. People having weak bones (osteoporosis) must have calcium and vitamin D.
   viii. People following 'fad' diets, engaging in multiple fasting days, adopting extreme dietary patterns or using major weight-loss drugs require appropriate guidance and monitoring for supplements. Vegetarians need more vitamin B_{12}.
   ix. Those with chronic alcohol consumption will need more vitamin B complex.

Adverse Effects of Dietary Supplements and Vitamins

1. High doses of beta-carotene (found in carrots [*gajar*], spinach [*paalak*], lettuce [*salad patta*], tomatoes [*tamatar*], sweet potatoes [*shakarakand*] and broccoli [*brokolee*]) have been associated with lung cancer in smokers.[1]
2. High doses of calcium and vitamin D may cause kidney stones. Vitamin D in high doses is toxic and causes a dangerous increase in blood calcium level.
3. A high amount of protein can damage kidneys in those who are predisposed to it, for example, people with a single kidney, a dysfunctional kidney or diabetes.[2]

4. Several supplements have been linked to liver damage.[2]
5. Contrary to usual belief, popping multiple vitamins does not improve health and may be detrimental. However, selected vitamins are necessary in patients with diabetes, especially if patients are not eating in a balanced manner or if there is a problem in intestinal absorption of vitamins. Sometimes, prescription of vitamins will depend on a specific condition presumed to be due to vitamin deficiency and based on blood vitamin levels.

Vitamin D: The 'Sunshine Hormone'

Vitamin D is important for bone metabolism and also plays a role in the normal functioning of skeletal muscles, the immune system and glucose metabolism. It is made in the skin upon exposure to sunshine. Recent studies from our group show that vitamin D supplementation helps to decrease blood sugar levels in people with vitamin D deficiency.[3]

Causes of Deficiency

1. Less exposure to direct sunlight due to the person remaining indoors and commuting by cars, buses or metro.
2. Decreased cutaneous synthesis due to darker skin pigmentation (particularly relevant to Indians).
3. Use of sun blocks and too much coverage of the body with clothes, particularly in women.

Symptoms

There may be no symptoms or the following symptoms may occur:

1. Bone and muscle pains
2. Fractures due to fragile bones even on slight impact
3. Short stature in children

Calcium

1. Calcium is an essential component of intracellular processes that occur within bones, skeletal muscles and fat.
2. Consuming enough calcium (between 1,000 and 1,200 mg per day) is important for healthy men and women. However, receiving higher amounts of calcium over a long period of

time raises the risk of kidney stones in some people. Dietary sources of calcium are given in Table 6.1.

3. Some studies show an association between low calcium and vitamin D levels and diabetes. Supplements that combine both calcium and vitamin D may, therefore, help improve blood sugar levels and insulin action in patients with diabetes,[4] but more research is required.
4. Contrary to popular belief, taking oral calcium does not lead to calcium deposition in arteries. However, excess and unnecessary calcium intake should be avoided.
5. Calcium should be taken according to physicians' advice, especially if the patient has kidney damage, parathyroid disorder or high blood calcium levels.

TABLE 6.1 Dietary Sources of Calcium

Food Category	High Calcium	Ca (mg)	Moderate Calcium	Ca (mg)	Low Calcium	Ca (mg)
Milk and milk products	Buffalo milk	210	Cow's milk	120	Human milk	28
	Curd (*dahi*) (cow's milk)	149	Goat's milk	170	Buttermilk (*chaach*)	30
	Chenna (cow's milk)	208	Skimmed milk	120		
	Cheese	790				
	Khoa (whole cow milk)	956				
	Khoa (skimmed milk)	990				
	Skimmed milk powder	1,370				
Cereal grains and products	Finger millet (*ragi*)	364	Whole-wheat flour (*atta*)	39	Maize (*makka*)	9
			Pearl millet (*bajra*)	28	Rice raw milled/ parboiled	8
					Rice flakes (*chiwra*)/ puffed rice (*murmura*)/ vermicelli (*sewiyan*)	9

Food Category	High Calcium	Ca (mg)	Moderate Calcium	Ca (mg)	Low Calcium	Ca (mg)
Pulses and legumes	Whole Bengal gram (*chana dal*)	150	Black gram dal (*kaala chana dal*)	55		
	Whole horse gram (*kulathi*)	287	Bengal gram dal	43		
	Moth beans	154	Cowpea (*lobia*)	81		
	Kidney beans (*rajma*)	134	Green gram whole (*moong dal*)	124		
	Soybean-brown	240	Lentils (*dal*)	69		
	Soybean-white	195				
Leafy vegetables	Fenugreek leaves (*methi*)	274	Goosefoot (*bathua*) leaves	211	Cauliflower greens (*phool gobhi ke patte*)	96
	Colocasia leaves (*arbi ke patte*)	460	Radish leaves (*mooli ke patte*)	234	Lettuce (*salad patta*)	56
	Knol-khol greens (*kadam ke patte*)	368	Mustard leaves (*sarson ke patte*)	191		
	Amaranth greens (*rajgeera*)	330	Spinach (*paalak*)	73		
			Cabbage (*patta gobhi*)	170		
			Mint leaves (*pudhina*)	205		
Roots and tubers	Ladies' finger (*bhindi*)	86	Yam	45	Potato (*aaloo*), brown skin, small	8
			Carrot (*gajar*)	35		
			Colocasia (*arbi*)	30		
Nuts and oil seeds	Almond (*badam*)	228	Groundnut (*moongphali*)	54		
	Gingelly (*til*) seeds (white)	1,283	Linseed/ flaxseeds (*alsi*)	257		
	Gingelly (*til*) seeds (black)	1,664	Pistachio (*pista*)	135		

Food Category	High Calcium	Ca (mg)	Moderate Calcium	Ca (mg)	Low Calcium	Ca (mg)
	Mustard (*sarson*)	402			Coconut dry	32
	Sunflower seeds (*sarson ke beej*)	280				
Meat and poultry			Egg (hen)	60		
Fish and sea foods			Catfish (*singhala*)	98	Rohu	40
			Sardine	90		
			Prawns	68		
			Catfish	61	Tuna	10

Note: All values are mg per 100 g of edible portion.
Source: ICMR-NIN Expert Committee[5]
Any differences in nutrient values reflect variations in data sources, analytical methods and preparation methods.

Deficiency of calcium leads to:

1. Easy fracturing of bones (osteoporosis)
2. Muscle cramps due to poor muscle function
3. Heart dysfunction
4. Memory loss

Vitamin B_{12}

1. Vitamin B_{12} is necessary for a healthy nervous system and healthy blood cells. The best way to get vitamin B_{12} is through the diet (Table 6.2).
2. This vitamin is low in the vegetarian population and those people who take non-vegetarian food infrequently.
3. Consuming sufficient vitamin B_{12} is not enough as it needs to be absorbed efficiently.
4. Use of metformin, which is usually the first-line treatment for diabetes, may cause deficiency of B_{12}.

TABLE 6.2 Dietary Sources of Vitamin B_{12}

Food Product	Vitamin B_{12} (µg)
1. Dairy Products	
Milk and Milk Products	
Milk (cow's milk)	0.14

Food Product	Vitamin B_{12} (μg)
Curd (*dahi*) (cow's milk)	0.13
Skimmed milk powder	0.8
Low-fat skimmed milk	0.5
Cheese (Swiss)	3.3
2. Flesh Foods	
Egg (hen, whole)	1.8
Egg white	0.2
Egg yolk (hen)	4.4
Mutton	2.6
Liver, goat	80–90
3. Fish	
Shrimp, fresh	9.0
Mackerel	19
Salmon	8

Note: All values are μg per 100 g of edible portion.
Source: Reproduced from *Diabetes with Delight* by Anoop Misra.[6]
Any differences in nutrient values reflect variations in data sources, analytical methods and preparation methods.

Vitamin B_{12} in Fortified Products

1. Fortified soy milk: Soy foods and soy 'meat' are a good food source of vitamin B_{12} if they are fortified. Fortified soy products per 100 g contain 2.4 μg of vitamin B_{12}.
2. Fortified cereals (all bran) per 100 g contain 20 μg of vitamin B_{12}.

Deficiency

Deficiency of B_{12} vitamin can cause the following:

1. Anaemia, which may cause weakness, tiredness and light-headedness
2. Palpitations and/or shortness of breath
3. Nerve-related problems such as numbness or tingling (mostly in the soles and feet, that is, neuropathy), muscle weakness and difficulty in walking
4. A smooth ('bald') tongue ('atrophic glossitis') and altered mouth
5. Constipation, diarrhoea and loss of appetite
6. Depression, memory loss and/or behavioural changes

Folic Acid (Vitamin B_9)

What Does Folic Acid Do to the Body?

1. It is required to synthesise nucleic acids, which are essential to body functions.
2. It aids in rapid cell division and growth.
3. It helps form red blood cells.
4. It is important for pregnant women to have enough folic acid to prevent major birth defects of the baby's brain or spine (neural tube defects, including spina bifida and anencephaly).
5. It helps to enhance brain health.

Deficiency

Deficiency of folic acid results in megaloblastic anaemia, which is often seen in children and pregnant women.

Foods with High Folic Acid Content

1. Beans (*phaliyan*) and lentils (*dal*)
2. Peas (*matar*), for example, black-eyed peas (*lobia*), chickpeas (*chole*) and green peas (*matar*)
3. Soy milk
4. Green leafy vegetables such as spinach (*paalak*), lettuce (*salad patta*), turnip greens (*shalgam*), mustard greens (*sarson ka saag*), cabbage (*patta gobhi*), broccoli (*brokolee*), corn (*makka*), cauliflower (*phool gobhi*), potato (*aaloo*) and green onions
5. Fortified foods (some brands of breakfast cereals, pasta, cornmeal, white rice, flour)

Potassium (K)

What Does Potassium Do to the Body?

1. Potassium is one of the most important electrolytes in the human body.
2. Potassium is vital for the healthy functioning of cells, tissues and organs. It helps to maintain a healthy blood pH level.
3. Potassium is particularly important for the ability of skeletal and smooth muscles to contract. It is vital to the health of the heart and for normal heart rhythm/heartbeats.

4. Dietary sources of potassium are given in Table 6.3.
5. Safe intake of potassium per day is 2,500 mg/day.
6. If you have damaged or impaired kidneys, potassium should be restricted to avoid developing an irregular heartbeat.
7. High potassium is bad for the heart, while low potassium causes weakness of muscles.
8. Kidney failure and some drugs used in treatment of blood pressure (angiotensin-converting enzyme inhibitors, angiotensin receptor blockers) can increase potassium levels.

TABLE 6.3 Dietary Sources of Potassium

Food Category	High Potassium	K (mg)	Moderate Potassium	K (mg)	Low Potassium	K (mg)
Fruits	Gooseberry (*amla*)	223	Musk melon (*kharbooja*)	196		
	Dried dates (*khajoor*)	782				
	Dry apricot (*sookha khubani*)	285	Apple (*seb*)	100		
	Guava (*amrood*)	285				
	Avocado (*makhanphal*)	377	Pomegranate (*anar*)	206		
	Raisins (*kishmish*)	1,105				
	Peach (*aadu*)	281	*Litchi*	161		
	Ripe banana (*paka kela*)	362		173		
	Pear (*nashpati*)	362	Plum (*aaloo bukara*)	162		
			Orange (*santra*)	164		
			Red cherries	165		
	Lemon (*nimbu*)	270				
	Ripe mango (*aam*)	205				
Pulses and legumes	Bengal gram (*chana dal*)	957				
	Horse gram (*kulathi*)	1,065				
	Moth beans (*moth*)	1,356				
	Kidney beans (*rajma*)	1,362				

Food Category	High Potassium	K (mg)	Moderate Potassium	K (mg)	Low Potassium	K (mg)
	Soybean	1,613				
	Whole lentils (*chilke vali dal*)	1,356				
	Cowpea (*lobia*)	1,241				
	Whole green gram (*moong sabut*)	1,117				
Leafy vegetables	Amaranth (*raj-geera*)	572				
	Cabbage (*patta gobhi*)	292				
	Coriander leaves (*dhania*)	256	Fenugreek leaves (*methi*)	226		
	Spinach (*paalak*)	625	Lettuce (*salad patta*)	279		
Roots and tubers	Colocasia (*arbi*)	550	Beetroot (*chukandar*)	43	Arrowroot flour	20
	Potato (*aaloo*)	247	Carrot (*gajar*)	108		
	Sweet potato (*shakarakand*)	343	Onion (*pyaz*)	127		
Other vegetables	Brinjal (*baingan*)	300	Radish (*mooli*)	138		
	Jackfruit (*kathal*)	327	Bitter gourd (*karela*)	326	Round gourd (*tinda*)	116
			Bottle gourd (*lauki*)	116		
	Cauliflower (*phool gobhi*)	329				
			Cucumber (*kheera*)	183		
			Ladies' finger (*bhindi*)	263		
	Pumpkin (*seetha phal*)	253	Ridge gourd (*tori*)	50		
Nuts and oils seeds	Almonds (*badam*)	699				
	Walnuts (*akhrot*)	457				
Milk and milk products	Cow's milk	115	Buffalo milk	109		
	Curd (*dahi*) (cow's milk)	130				
	Cottage cheese (*paneer non-fat*)	137				

Food Category	High Potassium	K (mg)	Moderate Potassium	K (mg)	Low Potassium	K (mg)
Cereal grain and products	Finger millet (*ragi*)	443	Semolina (*suji*)	83		
	Whole-wheat flour (*atta*)	366	Refined wheat flour (*maida*)	148		
	Pearl millet (*bajra*)	365				
	Rice flakes (*chiwra*)	148				

Note: All values are mg per 100 g of edible portion.
Source: ICMR-NIN Expert Committee[5]
Any differences in nutrient values reflect variations in data sources, analytical methods and preparation methods.

Easy Reading 16

A Colourful Approach to Eating with the New Indian Dietary Guidelines

The new dietary guidelines released by the National Institute of Nutrition have taken a commendable approach, employing visuals such as a plate featuring various healthy food groups on the first page and concluding with a detailed food pyramid on page 148.[6] Within these guidelines, comprehensive information is provided regarding healthy food choices, cooking techniques, the impact of processed foods and guidance on interpreting food labels.

While the majority of individuals are familiar with the three macronutrients—carbohydrates, fats and proteins—there is a need for further discussion on these topics. Carbohydrates, often regarded as the cornerstone of our diets, raise a fundamental question: What types of carbohydrates should we prioritise? Among them, whole grains such as millets, quinoa and oats (*jai*) are highlighted for their nutritional value, yet it's crucial to recognise their disparities. For instance, barley (*jau*) has a high fibre content and a low GI (denoting a lower rise in blood sugar after consumption), making it a favourable choice for individuals with obesity or diabetes. Conversely, finger millet (*ragi*) is rich in calcium, which is beneficial for those with dietary calcium needs, but its relatively high GI renders it less suitable for individuals with diabetes. Despite recent criticisms, wheat (*gehu*) remains a budget-friendly and nutritious option. A single medium-sized roti contains approximately 3 g fibre and 3.8 g protein. If one consumes four such *roti*s daily, they will fulfil about 12 g fibre (roughly one-third of the daily requirement) and 15 g of protein (equivalent to 26 percent of the daily protein requirement). It would be best to have wheat mixed with *jowar* or *besan* to have the least sugar excursions after meals. These insights, integral to the metabolically friendly needs of Indians, warrant discussion within the guidelines.

The graphics featured in the chapter discussing oils and fats are impeccably crafted, providing valuable guidance on the limitation (or even better, avoidance) of oils rich in saturated fats such as ghee, coconut oil, palm oil and butter. The bad effects of these oils are not limited to heart disease and stroke, as stated, but also fatty liver and liver damage, which we see widely today. The emphasis placed on 'good fats' like PUFAs found in nuts, seeds, soybeans, fish, grains, millets, green leafy vegetables and fenugreek is commendable as they are rightfully highlighted on the food plate. However, another category of beneficial fats, MUFAs, is equally, if not more, deserving of attention. These fats, present in oils such as mustard, olive and canola, as well as in almonds (*badam*), peanuts (*moongphali*), avocado (*makhanphal*) and the like, offer significant health benefits. Their inclusion in the dietary guidelines should be underscored to ensure a comprehensive understanding of optimal fat consumption.

One of the most well-articulated chapters in the dietary guidelines pertains to proteins. Indians require increased protein consumption for the development of muscle mass and metabolic health. Our food should contain about 15 percent of calories from protein sources (about 0.8 g/kg of body weight). The best distribution of protein is 25 percent with each major meal and the remaining 25 percent divided between two snacks. Interestingly, a protein snack before sleeping improves muscle building through the night. While there is often a tendency to turn to non-vegetarian sources (eggs, lean meats) for augmenting protein intake, the guidelines succinctly advocate for the combination of cereals (such as wheat and millets) with pulses (including lentils [*dal*], chickpeas [*chole*], green gram [*moong*], kidney beans [*rajma*]), soybeans, tofu and cowpeas (*lobia*) in a ratio of 3:1 to enhance protein quality. Specifically, whole eggs are a good form of protein, are easily available and should be consumed by all except those with markedly high cholesterol and heart disease. There is an increased need for protein in children, pregnant women (requiring an additional 8–18 g per day), older adults, individuals with chronic illnesses or cancer or those recovering from surgery or a significant infection of COVID-19. On the other hand, protein should be judiciously taken and even reduced in people with kidney disease or high uric acid levels.

This approach should provide enough protein from specified dietary sources, and extra protein supplements are not required. In this context, cautionary advice against the prolonged intake of protein supplements is well founded. However, statements such as the potential increase in the risk of certain non-communicable diseases due to the intake of branched-chain amino acids (essential proteins found in whey protein) should be tempered, as the evidence supporting such claims is not yet conclusive.

It is suggested that the committee could benefit from additional insights by including a clinician as a member. Additionally, dedicating a small paragraph in certain chapters to address dietary considerations for patients with diabetes and heart disease would enhance relevance. Furthermore, it is essential to include appropriate scientific references to support the information provided. The dissemination of the messages contained within these pages to the general population is crucial, and therefore, it is recommended to include easy-to-understand practical points specifically for laypersons to implement after each chapter.

These guidelines embody a significant endeavour, nicely crafted to engage and inform. They are well illustrated with graphics and tables, conveying the vital message of embracing diverse colours and a variety of fruits, vegetables, nuts, seeds and whole grains. One should ask: What is the colour of my diet? The answer lies in the concept of a 'rainbow diet,' akin to the colourful plate depicted on the very first page.

Note: This article was published on the following site: https://merotribune.com/2025/01/18/a-colorful-approach-to-eating-with-new-indian-guidelines/#:~:text=Our%20food%20should%20incorporate%20about,muscle%20building%20through%20the%20night

Easy Reading 17

Vitamins and Supplements: Good for a Selected Few?

Dietary supplements are available in pure forms (for example, vitamin B_{12}, fish oil, vitamin D and whey protein) and mixed together (multivitamins include a few to thirty or more vitamins and minerals together). The latter is consumed widely.

We see all kinds of misuse of vitamins and supplements. A sixty-year-old gentleman consulted me about his loss of appetite. On questioning, he showed me a list of seventeen supplements (written on a scrap of worn-out paper) that he was taking. These ranged from vitamins and hormones to steroids. He said that he just wanted to live longer than others by consuming these 'energy-giving supplements'. Investigations revealed a frayed liver (high liver enzymes indicating liver damage), and urine showed plenty of proteins (indicating kidney damage). I told him; 'By consuming this dangerous cocktail of supplements and hormones, you may live shorter than others.' I stopped all his supplements, and his liver and kidneys gradually healed.

Another patient came to me with very high calcium levels, which was causing kidney failure. On questioning, he said, 'I had heard that all of us have vitamin D deficiency, so I started taking it daily. He bought it over the counter and, without a physician's advice, took one sachet of 60,000 units of vitamin D daily for the last three months (meant to be taken once weekly for a limited time in those with vitamin D deficiency). He was admitted to the hospital, and we were able to bring down the calcium level gradually. Then, his kidney function improved.

The lesson is that you do not need vitamins and minerals if you are without any disease, exercising regularly and taking nutritious diets that include plenty of fruits and vegetables. Enough vitamins/minerals could be acquired from the following sources: vitamin D from sunshine exposure; calcium from milk, curds (*dahi*) and cheese; B_{12} from liver and seafood, etc.; and protein from non-vegetarian sources, soybean, milk, nuts, Bengal gram, lentils (*dal*), flaxseeds (*alsi*) and so on.

Which condition requires supplements? A patient should be guided by a doctor or a nutritionist. When food absorption is decreased in the intestine (malabsorption, pancreatic inflammation or intestinal surgery), several vitamins become deficient. Patients who have lost a lot of weight (cancer, liver disease and the like) will require vitamin and protein supplements. Those who take a considerable amount of alcohol for long periods become deficient in vitamins. Those with fragile bones and thin muscles require vitamins, calcium and protein supplements. Iron supplements are needed in several conditions: heavy periods in women, intestinal ulcers, worm infestations and so on. Remember, multiple deficiencies of vitamins and protein may occur after any acute infections (viral or bacterial), and this has been seen to occur in a severe manner in those with COVID-19 infections. Pregnant women clearly need vitamins to prevent birth defects from occurring in offspring. Some vegetarian people may suffer from vitamin B_{12} and protein deficiency. In alcohol withdrawal, thiamine supplementation becomes necessary.

Patients with diabetes are often prescribed multivitamins. Those on commonly prescribed drugs such as metformin will need vitamin B_{12}. Those with long-standing diabetes, who are frail and have poor appetite or intestinal muscle dysfunction (due to severe nerve damage) will need multivitamin and vitamin D supplements. Protein supplements should be given with great care in patients having kidney dysfunction. Patients with diabetes often have high blood fats (triglycerides), and these could be effectively treated by fish oil capsules (made from oils of salmon and other fatty fishes).

Young men who want to build their muscles are given protein supplements in gyms. These may help; however, the dose of total protein intake needs to be calculated properly according to body weight. Other additions such as body-building hormones (anabolic steroids) should be avoided. These supplements are given in many gyms by unqualified people.

Like excess vitamin D (refer to the second patient mentioned earlier) and calcium, intake of some other vitamins may also cause harm. Avoid beta-carotene (from pills, but it is fine from natural foods) if you are a smoker/ex-smoker and vitamin A if you are pregnant. Excess vitamin E taken for long periods may increase the risk for prostate cancer.

Some people think that if they are taking one multivitamin tablet, they will have enough of all vitamins and minerals. That is not true. Specific vitamin/mineral deficiencies (vitamin B_{12}, folate, calcium, iron, vitamin D and so on) need to be treated with pure specific vitamins/minerals (tailored therapy), which are given in 5–10 times higher doses than found in a multivitamin capsule/tablet. In severe deficiency, injectable vitamins need to be given.

Finally, there is a misconception that taking daily vitamins/minerals will prevent heart disease or cancer. There is no evidence that this will take place in those who are taking a variety of healthy diets, fruits and vegetables and going out in sunlight to do aerobic exercise. Clearly, a multivitamin a day cannot replace a healthy diet and exercise.

Note: This article, originally featured in *The Indian Express*, has been revised and updated from its initial published version.

Easy Reading 18

Hidden Nutrients: Important for Patients with Diabetes and for Older Adults

The relative of a seventy-eight-year-old patient with multiple diseases, including diabetes, asked me: 'What are the nutrients required for my father?' I stated, 'At this age and with multiple diseases, both nutrients and micronutrients are important. Importantly, these must be given judiciously.' Then I explained to him in the following manner.

There are three macronutrients: protein, carbohydrates and fats. These are essential for health and need to be taken in the right proportion. These are visible and relatively large in quantity in food. On the other hand, micronutrients are plentiful and present in various foods in a very small amount and often cannot be seen with the eyes. Deficiencies of micronutrients are substantial in people living in developing countries like India and much less in Western countries.

There are several micronutrients, such as iron, vitamins (B_{12}, other B vitamins, folate, vitamin D, vitamin A, vitamin C), minerals (magnesium, calcium, selenium), iodine, sodium, potassium, chloride, sulphur and so on. The classical example of a severe micronutrient deficiency is scurvy. This used to occur in sea-bound people who did not eat fruits (a source of vitamin C) for several days and suffered from bleeding in their gums and at other places. Such extreme deficiencies are rare now. However, even slight deficiencies of some micronutrients could disturb organ functions and smooth functioning of the body. Enough daily intake to avoid deficiencies is termed as recommended dietary allowances (RDA). Several diseases occur due to micronutrient deficiencies: goitre due to iodine deficiency, anaemia due to iron deficiency, nerve damage due to vitamin B deficiency, rickets/bone weakness due to vitamin D/calcium deficiency, anaemia/foetal damage due to folate deficiency and so on.

In India, deficiency of iron, vitamin D, vitamin B_{12} and iodine is widespread. These deficiencies occur more commonly in the following situations: childhood, adolescence, pregnancy and old age. Deficiencies may also occur in stressful situations such as fever, long illnesses, intestinal dysfunctions leading to malabsorption, chronic bleeding, diarrhoea, vomiting and chronic kidney and liver diseases. Deficiencies of micronutrients in growing age or pregnancy may impact development of the brain, bones, immunity, blood clotting and other vital organ functions.

Patients with diabetes may have micronutrient deficiency, particularly those who have uncontrolled blood sugar and suffer from complications. Interestingly, our research shows that vitamin D deficiency may have a role in diabetes control and that it should be corrected by giving supplements. A main drug for diabetes, metformin, when used in high doses and for a long time will result in vitamin B_{12} deficiency. In such cases, vitamin B_{12} supplementation is required. Interestingly, multiple deficiencies are seen in patients with diabetes who are lacto-vegetarians (B_{12}, iodine, zinc) and vegans (iron, zinc, folate, B_{12}, iodine). There is the emerging role of magnesium in regulation of blood sugar as well.

Older adults suffer from multiple micronutrient deficiencies due to insufficient food intake, intestinal dysfunction, dental problems, multiple illnesses and so on. One study showed that 20–60 percent of older adults would have one or more such deficiencies, and this figure could be higher in India. They should be carefully evaluated for both macro- (mostly protein) and micronutrient deficits. Besides balancing foods, most such individuals will need multiple vitamins and minerals to correct these deficits. Sometimes injectable therapy is needed (for example, iron, vitamin B_{12}, vitamin D). Frequent and prolonged use of antiacid medications (pantoprazole, omeprazole) in older adults (or for that matter anybody) could lead to vitamin B_{12}, vitamin C, calcium and magnesium deficiencies.

Pills that have multiple vitamins and minerals are commonly sold over the counter. Many people pop these pills without their physicians' supervision. In some cases, these may help, but in most cases of micronutrient deficiencies, they do not. In those with major vitamin and mineral deficiencies, high doses of specific nutrients are necessary (for example, vitamin D, B_{12}). Specific vitamins like folate are required in pregnancy to avoid birth defects. Finally, supplementation of these vitamins and minerals is not without toxic effects as seen in excess doses of vitamin D, zinc, calcium and the like. Patients with diabetes and kidney disease, when given excess potassium (mostly in fruits), develop life-threatening heart irregularities. Hence, these important small nutrients must be taken under expert observation.

Note: This article, originally featured in *The Indian Express*, has been revised and updated from its initial published version.

Acknowledgements

I would like to express my hearty thanks to Bhavya Arora for her meticulous editing of this book and for her invaluable advice throughout the writing process.

This work is built upon a foundation of rigorous science, and I am deeply thankful to all the members of my research and clinical teams. Without their dedication and hard work, I would not have been able to present the robust research data that defines this book. It is their collective effort that ensures these pages are based on evidence specifically generated for and applicable to Indian patients.

Lastly, I am profoundly indebted to my patients. Over the years, they have been my greatest teachers, providing the insights and experiences that have truly shaped my understanding of health and nutrition.

References

Chapter 1 What Is a Healthy Diet?

1 WHO. Healthy diets [cited 2025 Mar]. Available from: https://www.who.int/health-topics/healthy-diet#tab=tab_1.

2 National Institute of Diabetes and Digestive and Kidney Diseases. Diet and nutrition [cited 2025 Mar]. Available from: https://www.niddk.nih.gov/health-information/diet-nutrition.

3 Center for Disease Control and Prevention (CDC). About nutrition [cited 2025 Mar]. Available from: https://www.cdc.gov/nutrition/php/about/index.html.

4 ICMR-NIN Expert Committee. ICMR NIN dietary guidelines for Indians. Hyderabad: ICMR, National Institute of Nutrition; 2024 [cited 2025 Mar]. Available from: https://main.icmr.nic.in/sites/default/files/upload_documents/DGI_07th_May_2024_fin.pdf.

Chapter 2 Basics of Diets

1 Anoop Misra. *Diabetes with Delight*. New Delhi: Bloomsbury India; 2018.

2 Longvah T, Ananthan R, Bhaskarachary K, Venkaiah K. *Indian food composition tables.* Hyderabad, Telangana: National Institute of Nutrition Indian [Council of Medical Research]; 2017 [cited 2025 Mar]. Available from: https://www.nin.res.in/ebooks/IFCT2017.pdf.

3 United States Department of Agriculture. FoodData Central: SR legacy foods [Internet]. Washington (DC): USDA; [cited 2025 Oct]. Available from: https://fdc.nal.usda.gov/food-search?type=SR%20Legacy&query=protein.

4 Mohan V, Misra A, Bhansali A, *et al.* Role and significance of dietary protein in the management of type 2 diabetes and its complications in India: an expert opinion. *J Assoc Physicians India*. 2023 Dec;71(12):36–46. doi:10.59556/japi.71.0339.

5 Saboo B, Misra A, Kalra S, *et al.* Role and importance of high fiber in diabetes management in India. *Diabetes Metab Syndr.* 2022 May;16(5):102480. doi: 10.1016/j.dsx.2022.102480.

Chapter 3 Current Dietary Trends, Diabetes Reversal and Weight Loss Options

1 Kirkpatrick KW, Bolick JP, Kris-Etherton PM, *et al.* Review of current evidence and clinical recommendations on the effects of low-carbohydrate and very-low-carbohydrate (including ketogenic) diets for the management of body weight and other cardiometabolic risk factors: a scientific statement from the National Lipid Association Nutrition and Lifestyle Task Force. *J Clin Lipidol.* 2019 Sep-Oct;13(5):689-711.e1. doi: 10.1016/j.jacl.2019.08.003.

2 Kosinski C, Jornayvaz FR. Effects of ketogenic diets on cardiovascular risk factors: evidence from animal and human studies. *Nutrients* 2017 May 19;9(5):517. doi: 10.3390/nu9050517.

3 American College of Cardiology. 'Keto-like' diet may be linked to higher risk of heart disease, cardiac events. Press release, 2023 Mar 5 [cited 2005 Feb]. Available from: https://www.acc.org/About-ACC/Press-Releases/2023/03/05/15/07/Keto-Like-Diet-May-Be-Linked-to-Higher-Risk.

4 Latan I, Huang K, Vikulova D, *et al.* Association of a low-carbohydrate high-fat diet with plasma lipid levels and cardiovascular risk. *JACC Adv.* 2024 Mar 25;3(6):100924. doi:10.1016/j.jacadv.2024.100924. eCollection 2024 Jun. PMID: 39081652.

5 Zhu H, Bi D, Zhang Y, *et al.* Ketogenic diet for human diseases: the underlying mechanisms and potential for clinical implementations. *Signal Transduct Target Ther.* 2022 Jan 17;7(1):11. doi: 10.1038/s41392-021-00830-x.

6 Patikorn C, Saidoung P, Pham T, *et al.* Effects of ketogenic diet on health outcomes: an umbrella review of meta-analyses of randomized clinical trials. *BMC Med.* 2023 May 25;21(1):196. doi: 10.1186/s12916-023-02874-y.

7 Yang F, Liu C, Liu X, *et al.* Effect of epidemic intermittent fasting on cardiometabolic risk factors: a systematic review and meta-analysis of randomized controlled trials. *Front Nutr.* 2021 Oct 18;8:669325. doi:10.3389/fnut.2021.669325.

8 Semnani-Azad Z, Khan TA, Chiavaroli L, *et al.* Intermittent fasting strategies and their effects on body weight and other cardiometabolic risk factors: systematic review and network meta-analysis of randomised clinical trials. *BMJ.* 2025;389:e082007.

9 Halpern B, Mendes TB. Intermittent fasting for obesity and related disorders: unveiling myths, facts, and presumptions. *Arch Endocrinol Metab.* 2021 Nov 1;65(1):14–23. doi:10.20945/2359-3997000000322.

10 Chen M, Xu L, Van Horn L, *et al.* Association of eating duration less than 8 h with all-cause, cardiovascular, and cancer mortality.

Diabetes Metab Syndr. 2025;In Press:103278. doi:10.1016/j.dsx.2025.103278.

11 Misra A, Gupta R, *et al.* Intermittent fasting: evidence for benefit, lack of effect, or potential cardiometabolic risk? *Diabetes Metab Syndr.* 2025;In Press:103280. doi:10.1016/j.dsx.2025.103280.

12 Carter S, Clifton PM, Keogh JB. Effect of intermittent compared with continuous energy-restricted diet on glycemic control in patients with type 2 diabetes: a randomized noninferiority trial. *JAMA Netw Open.* 2018 Jul 6;1(3):e180756. doi: 10.1001/jamanetworkopen.2018.0756. PMID: 30646030.

13 Oldenburg N, Mashek DG, Harnack L, *et al.* Time-restricted eating, caloric reduction, and unrestricted eating effects on weight and metabolism: a randomized trial. *Obesity (Silver Spring).* 2025 Feb 19. doi: 10.1002/oby.24252.

14 Lowe DA, Wu N, Rohdin-Bibby N, *et al.* Effects of time-restricted eating on weight loss and other metabolic parameters in women and men with overweight and obesity: the TREAT randomized clinical trial. *JAMA Intern Med* 2020 Sep 28;180(11):1-9. doi: 10.1001/jamainternmed.2020.415.

15 Sun ML, Yao W, Wang XY, *et al.* Intermittent fasting and health outcomes: an umbrella review of systematic reviews and meta-analyses of randomised controlled trials. *EClinicalMedicine.* 2024 Apr;70:102519. doi: 10.1016/j.eclinm.2024.102519.

16 Yao K, Su H, Cui K, *et al.* Effectiveness of an intermittent fasting diet versus regular diet on fat loss in overweight and obese middle-aged and elderly people without metabolic disease: a systematic review and meta-analysis of randomized controlled trials. *J Nutr Health Aging.* 2024 Mar;28(3):100165. doi: 10.1016/j.jnha.2024.100165. Epub 2024 Feb 2. PMID: 38308923.

17 Patikorn C, Roubal K, Veettil SK, *et al.* Intermittent fasting and obesity-related health outcomes: an umbrella review of meta-analyses of randomized clinical trials. *JAMA Netw Open.* 2021 Dec 1;4(12):e2139558. doi:10.1001/jamanetworkopen.2021.

18 Elias A, Padinjakara N, Lautenschlager NT. Effects of intermittent fasting on cognitive health and Alzheimer's disease. *Nutr Rev.* 2023 Aug 10;81(9):1225–33. doi:10.1093/nutrit/nuad021. PMID: 37043764.

19 Selinger E, Neuenschwander M, Koller A, *et al.* Evidence of a vegan diet for health benefits and risks: an umbrella review of meta-analyses of observational and clinical studies. *Crit Rev Food Sci Nutr.* 2023;63(29):9926-36. doi: 10.1080/10408398.2022.2075311. Epub 2022 May 16.

20 Dinu M, Abbate R, Gensini GF, *et al.* Vegetarian, vegan diets and multiple health outcomes: a systematic review with meta-analysis

of observational studies. *Crit Rev Food Sci Nutr* 2017 Nov 22; 57(17):3640-9. doi: 10.1080/10408398.2016.1138447.

21 Benatar, J, Steward AH. Cardiometabolic risk factors in vegans; a meta-analysis of observational studies. *PLoS One*; 2018 Dec 20;13(12):e0209086.doi:10.1371/journal.pone.0209086.eCollection 2018.

22 Bakaloudi DR, Halloran A, Rippin HL, *et al.* Intake and adequacy of the vegan diet: a systematic review of the evidence. *Clin Nutr.* 2021 May;40(5):3503-21. doi: 10.1016/j.clnu.2020.11.035. Epub 2020 Dec 7. PMID: 33341313.

23 Lim EL, Hollingsworth KG, Aribisala BS, *et al.* Reversal of type 2 diabetes: normalisation of beta cell function in association with decreased pancreas and liver triacylglycerol. *Diabetologia.* 2011 Oct;54(10):2506-14. doi: 10.1007/s00125-011-2204-7.

24 Al-Mrabeh A, Hollingsworth KG, Shaw JAM, *et al.* 2-year remission of type 2 diabetes and pancreas morphology: a post-hoc analysis of the DiRECT open-label, cluster-randomised trial. *Lancet Diabetes Endocrinol.* 2020 Dec;8(12):939–48. doi: 10.1016/S2213-8587(20)30303-X.

25 Lean MEJ, Leslie WS, Barnes AC, *et al.* Primary care-led weight management for remission of type 2 diabetes (DiRECT): an open-label, cluster-randomised trial. *Lancet.* 2018 Feb 10;391(10120):541-51. doi: 10.1016/S0140-6736(17)33102-1. Epub 2017 Dec 5. PMID: 29221645.

26 Lean MEJ, Leslie WS, Barnes AC, *et al.* 5-year follow-up of the randomised Diabetes Remission Clinical Trial (DiRECT) of continued support for weight loss maintenance in the UK: an extension study. *Lancet Diabetes Endocrinol.* 2024 Apr;12(4):233-46. doi: 10.1016/S2213-8587(23)00385-6. Epub 2024 Feb 26. PMID: 38423026.

27 Kanbour S, Ageeb RA, Malik RA, *et al.* Impact of bodyweight loss on type 2 diabetes remission: a systematic review and meta-regression analysis of randomised controlled trials. *Lancet Diabetes Endocrinol.* 2025 Apr;13(4):294-306. doi: 10.1016/S2213-8587(24)00346-2. Epub 2025 Feb 26. PMID: 40023186.

28 Shamanna P, Joshi S, Shah L, *et al.* Type 2 diabetes reversal with digital twin technology-enabled precision nutrition and staging of reversal: a retrospective cohort study. *Clin Diabetes Endocrinol.* 2021;7:21. doi:10.1186/s40842-021-00134-7.

29 Heymsfield SB. Meal replacements and energy balance. *Physiol Behav.* 2010 Apr 26;100(1):90-4. doi: 10.1016/j.physbeh.2010.02.010. Epub 2010 Mar 1.

30 Yan M, Hu Y, Yin W, *et al.* The effect of total and partial meal replacements on obesity: a systematic review and meta-analysis of randomized controlled trials. *Crit Rev Food Sci Nutr.* 2025 Feb 28:1-9. doi: 10.1080/10408398.2025.2465768.

31 Gulati S, Misra A, Tiwari R, *et al.* Effect of high-protein meal replacement on weight and cardiometabolic profile in overweight/obese Asian Indians in North India. *Br J Nutr.* 2017 Jun;117(11):1531–40. doi: 10.1017/S0007114517001295.

32 Bhardwaj S, Misra A, Gulati S, *et al.* A randomized controlled trial to evaluate the effects of high-protein complete (lacto) vegetarian (PACER) diet in non-diabetic obese Asian Indians in North India. *Heliyon.* 2017 Dec;3(12):e00472. doi: 10.1016/j.heliyon.2017.e00472.

33 El Khoury D, Balfour-Ducharme S, Joye IJ. A review on the gluten-free diet: technological and nutritional challenges. *Nutrients.* 2018 Oct 2;10(10):1410. doi: 10.3390/nu10101410.

34 Lebwohl B, Cao Y, Zong G, *et al.* Long-term gluten consumption in adults without celiac disease and risk of coronary heart disease: prospective cohort study. *BMJ.* 2017 May 2;357:j1892. doi: 10.1136/bmj.j1892.

35 Zong G, Lebwohl B, Hu FB, *et al.* Gluten intake and risk of type 2 diabetes in three large prospective cohort studies of US men and women. *Diabetologia.* 2018 Aug 3;61(10):2164-73. doi: 10.1007/s00125-018-4697-9. PMCID: PMC6182774.

36 Uhde M, Bercik P, Moayyedi P, Armstrong D, Vanner S, *et al.* Symptomatic responses to #wheat, #gluten, and #gluten-free sham in irritable bowel syndrome: a randomised, double-blind, sham-controlled crossover trial. *Lancet Gastroenterol Hepatol.* 2023;8(12):1120–31. doi:10.1016/S2468-1253(23)00303-2.

37 Borghini R, Spagnuolo A, Donato G, *et al.* Gluten-free diet for fashion or necessity? Review with new speculations on irritable bowel syndrome-like disorders. *Nutrients.* 2024 Dec 8;16(23):4236. doi: 10.3390/nu16234236. PMID: 39683629.

38 Niland B, Cash BD. Health benefits and adverse effects of a gluten-free diet in non-celiac disease patients. *Gastroenterol Hepatol (NY).* 2018 Feb;14(2):82-91.

39 National Geographic [Internet]. This island unlocked the secret to long life—and knows how to get through tough times. 2020 Oct 12 [cited 2025 Mar]; Available from: https://www.nationalgeographic.com/premium/article/uncover-the-secrets-of-longevity-in-this-japanese-village.

40 Gonzalez-Freire M, Diaz-Ruiz A, Hauser D, *et al.* The road ahead for health and lifespan interventions. *Ageing Res Rev.* 2020

May;59:101037. doi: 10.1016/j.arr.2020.101037. Epub 2020 Feb 25. PMID: 32109604.

41 Li S, Vazquez JM, Sudmant PH. The evolution of aging and lifespan. *Trends Genet.* 2023 Nov;39(11):830-43. doi: 10.1016/j.tig.2023.08.005. Epub 2023 Sep 14.

42 Gudzune KA, Kushner RF. Medications for obesity: a review. *JAMA.* 2024 Aug 20;332(7):571-584. doi: 10.1001/jama.2024.10816.

43 Chakhtoura M, Haber R, Ghezzawi M, *et al.* Pharmacotherapy of obesity: an update on the available medications and drugs under investigation. *EClinicalMedicine.* 2023 Mar 20;58:101882. doi: 10.1016/j.eclinm.2023.101882. eCollection 2023 Apr.

44 Perkovic V, Tuttle KR, Rossing P, *et al.* Effects of semaglutide on chronic kidney disease in patients with type 2 diabetes. *N Engl J Med.* 2024;391:109–21. doi:10.1056/NEJMoa2403347.

45 Malhotra A, Grunstein RR, Fietze I, *et al.* Tirzepatide for the treatment of obstructive sleep apnea and obesity. *N Engl J Med.* 2024;391:1193–1205. doi:10.1056/NEJMoa2404881.

46 Aronne LJ, Horn DB, le Roux CW, *et al.* Tirzepatide as compared with semaglutide for the treatment of obesity. *N Engl J Med.* 2025 May 11.

Chapter 4 Diets in Various Diseases and Conditions

1 Sekher TV, Flood D, Green H, *et al.* Prevalence, awareness, treatment, and control of diabetes in India: a nationally representative survey of adults aged 45 years and older. *Lancet Glob Health.* 2025 Sep;13(9):e1543-e1552. doi:10.1016/S2214-109X(23)00502-8. Epub 2025 Aug 7.

2 Anoop Misra. *Diabetes with Delight.* New Delhi: Bloomsbury India; 2018.

3 Chawla R, Madhu SV, Makkar BM, *et al.*, on behalf of the RSSDI-ESI Consensus Group. RSSDI-ESI clinical practice recommendations for the management of type 2 diabetes mellitus 2020. *Int J Diabetes Dev Ctries.* 2020 [cited 2025 Feb];40(Suppl 1):S1–S122. Available from: https://rssdi.in/newwebsite/pdfdata/Chawla2020_Article_RSSDI-ESI%20Clinical%20Practice%20Recom.pdf.

4 Mohan V, Misra A, Bhansali A, *et al.* Role and significance of dietary protein in the management of type 2 diabetes and its complications in India: an expert opinion. *J Assoc Physicians India.* 2023 Dec;71(12):36–46. doi: 10.59556/japi.71.0339.

5 Mohammad R, Bansod DW. Hypertension in India: a gender-based study of prevalence and associated risk factors. *BMC Public Health.* 2024;24:2681. doi:10.1186/s12889-024-20338-2.

6 Trumbo PR, Ard J, Bellisle F, *et al.* Perspective: current scientific evidence and research strategies in the role of almonds in cardiometabolic health. *Curr Dev Nutr.* 2024 Nov 28;9(1):104516. doi:10.1016/j.cdnut.2024.104516. eCollection 2025 Jan.

7 Adamczak M, Wiecek A. Food products that may cause an increase in blood pressure. *Curr Hypertens Rep.* 2020 Jan;22(1):2. doi: 10.1007/s11906-019-1007-y.

8 Appel LJ, Moore TJ, Obarzanek E, *et al.* A clinical trial of the effects of dietary patterns on blood pressure. *N Engl J Med.* 1997 Apr 17;336(16):1117-24. doi: 10.1056/NEJM199704173361601.

9 Ndanuko RN, Tapsell LC, Charlton KE, *et al.* Dietary patterns and blood pressure in adults: a systematic review and meta-analysis of randomized controlled trials. *Adv Nutr.* 2016 Jan 15;7(1):76-89. doi: 10.3945/an.115.009753.

10 Kim S, Jeong HN, Choi-Kwon S. The blood pressure control effect of the sodium-restricted Dietary Approaches to Stop Hypertension diet: a systematic review. *Br J Nutr.* 2024 Jul 28;132(2):141–50. doi:10.1017/S000711452400103X.

11 de Carvalho GB, Dias-Vasconcelos NL, Santos RKF, *et al.* Effect of different dietary patterns on glycemic control in individuals with type 2 diabetes mellitus: a systematic review. *Crit Rev Food Sci Nutr.* 2020;60(12):1999–2010. doi:10.1080/10408398.2019.

12 Quan X, Shen X, Li C, *et al.* Adherence to the Dietary Approaches to Stop Hypertension diet reduces the risk of diabetes mellitus: a systematic review and dose-response meta-analysis. *Endocrine.* 2024 Oct;86(1):85–100. doi:10.1007/s12020-024-03882-5. PMID: 38816664.

13 Bensaaud A, Seery S, Gibson I, *et al.* Dietary Approaches to Stop Hypertension (DASH) for the primary and secondary prevention of cardiovascular diseases. *Cochrane Database Syst Rev.* 2025 May 6;5(5):CD013729. doi:10.1002/14651858.CD013729.pub2.

14 Tan J, Wang C, Tomiyama AJ. Dietary Approaches to Stop Hypertension (DASH) diet and mental well-being: a systematic review. *Nutr Rev.* 2023 Dec 11;82(1):60–75. doi:10.1093/nutrit/nuad038. PMID: 37085157.

15 Abbasi MM, Babaahmadi P, Nozari F, *et al.* Association between adhering to a Dietary Approach to Stop Hypertension and risk of colorectal cancer: a systematic review and meta-analysis. *BMC Gastroenterol.* 2025 May 6;25(1):335. doi:10.1186/s12876-025-03859-2. PMID: 40329201.

16 Misra A, Kumar A, Kuchay MS, *et al.* Consensus guidelines for the diagnosis and management of metabolic dysfunction-associated

steatotic liver disease in adult Asian Indians with type 2 diabetes. *Diabetes Metab Syndr.* 2025;19(3):103209. doi:10.1016/j.dsx.2025.103209.

17 Bhatt SP, Misra A, Nigam P, *et al.* Nutrition and physical activity in Asian Indians with non-alcoholic fatty liver: a case-control study. *Diabetes Metab Syndr.* 2019 Mar-Apr;13(2):1271-4. doi: 10.1016/j.dsx.2019.01.054.

18 Hadefi A, Arvanitakis M, Trépo E, *et al.* Dietary strategies in non-alcoholic fatty liver disease patients: from evidence to daily clinical practice, a systematic review. *United European Gastroenterol J.* 2023 Sep;11(7):663-89. doi: 10.1002/ueg2.12443. Epub 2023 Jul 25.

19 Misra A, Kumar A, Kuchay MS, *et al.* Consensus guidelines for the diagnosis and management of metabolic dysfunction-associated steatotic liver disease in adult Asian Indians with type 2 diabetes. *Diabetes Metab Syndr.* 2025 Mar 5;19(3):103209. doi:10.1016/j.dsx.2025.103209. Online ahead of print.

20 Curtis E, Litwic A, Cooper C, *et al.* Determinants of muscle and bone aging. *J Cell Physiol.* 2015 Nov;230(11):2618-25. doi: 10.1002/jcp.25001.

21 Pal R, Aggarwal A, Singh T, *et al.* Diagnostic cut-offs, prevalence, and biochemical predictors of sarcopenia in healthy Indian adults: The Sarcopenia-Chandigarh Urban Bone Epidemiological Study (Sarco-CUBES). *Eur Geriatr Med.* 2020;11(5):725-36. doi:10.1007/s41999-020-00332-z.

22 Lonnie M, Hooker E, Brunstrom JM, *et al.* Protein for life: review of optimal protein intake, sustainable dietary sources and the effect on appetite in ageing adults. *Nutrients.* 2018 Mar 16;10(3):360. doi: 10.3390/nu10030360.

23 Mohan V, Misra A, Bhansali A, *et al.* Role and significance of dietary protein in the management of type 2 diabetes and its complications in India: an expert opinion. *J Assoc Physicians India.* 2023 Dec;71(12):36–46. doi:10.59556/japi.71.0339.

24 Pappas A, Liakou A, Zouboulis CC. Nutrition and skin. *Rev Endocr Metab Disord.* 2016 Sep;17(3):443-8.

25 Cicero AFG, Colletti A. Effects of carotenoids on health: are all the same? results from clinical trials. *Curr Pharm Des.* 2017; 23(17):2422-7. doi: 10.2174/1381612823666170207095459.

26 Ueda S, Tanahashi M, Higaki Y, *et al.* Ingestion of coffee polyphenols improves a scaly skin surface and the recovery rate of skin temperature after cold stress: a randomized, controlled trial. *J Nutr Sci Vitaminol* (Tokyo). 2017;63(5):291-7. doi: 10.3177/jnsv.63.291.

27 Duo L, Yang J, Wang X, *et al.* Krill oil: nutraceutical potential in skin health and disease. *Front Nutr.* 2024 Jul 12;11:1388155. doi: 10.3389/fnut.2024.1388155.

28 Vaughn AR, Sivamani RK. Effects of fermented dairy products on skin: a systematic review. *J Altern Complement Med*. 2015 Jul;21(7):380-5. doi: 10.1089/acm.2014.0261. Epub 2015 Jun 10.

29 Catalano A, Ceramella J, Iacopetta D, *et al.* Aloe vera—an extensive review focused on recent studies. *Foods*. 2024 Jul 8;13(13):2155. doi: 10.3390/foods13132155.

30 Agrawal AC, Garg AK. Epidemiology of osteoporosis. *Indian J Orthop.* 2023;57(Suppl 1):45-8. doi:10.1007/s43465-023-01012-3.

31 Sahni S, Mangano KM, McLean RR, *et al.* Dietary approaches for bone health: lessons from the Framingham Osteoporosis Study. *Curr Osteoporos Rep*. 2015 Aug;13(4):245-55. doi: 10.1007/s11914-015-0272-1.

32 Rizzoli R, Chevalley T, *et al.* Nutrition and osteoporosis prevention. *Curr Osteoporos Rep*. 2024 Dec;22(6):515-22. doi: 10.1007/s11914-024-00892-0.

33 Wallace TC. Dried plums, prunes and bone health: a comprehensive review. *Nutrients*. 2017 Apr 19;9(4):401. doi: 10.3390/nu9040401.

34 Price CT, Langford JR, Liporace FA, *et al.* Essential nutrients for bone health and a review of their availability in the average North American diet. *Open Orthop J*. 2012;6:143-9. doi: 10.2174/1874325001206010143.

35 Allen MS, Walter EE. Health-related lifestyle factors and sexual dysfunction: a meta-analysis of population-based research. *J Sex Med*. 2018 Apr;15(4):458-75. doi: 10.1016/j.jsxm.2018.02.008. Epub2018 Mar 6.

36 La J, Roberts NH, Yafi FA. Diet and men's sexual health. *Sex Med Rev.* 2018; 6:54-68.

37 Moran L, Brinkworth GD, Martin S, *et al.* Long-term effects of a randomised controlled trial comparing high protein or high carbohydrate weight loss diets on testosterone, SHBG, erectile and urinary function in overweight and obese men. *PLoS One*. 2016;11(9): e0161297. doi: 10.1371/journal.pone.0161297.

38 Salas-Huetos A, Muralidharan J, Galiè S, *et al.* Effect of nut consumption on erectile and sexual function in healthy males: a secondary outcome analysis of the FERTINUTS randomized controlled trial. *Nutrients*. 2019;11(6):1372. doi: 10.3390/nu11061372.

39 Cassidy A, Franz M, Rimm E. Dietary flavonoid intake and incidence of erectile dysfunction. *Am J Clin Nutr*. 2016;103(2):534–41. doi:10.3945/ajcn.115.122010.

40 Bauer SR, Breyer BJ, Stampfer MJ, *et al.* Association of diet with erectile dysfunction among men in the Health Professionals Follow-up Study. *JAMA Netw Open*. 2020;3(11):e2021701. doi:10.1001/jamanetworkopen.2020.21701.

41 Ghorbani Z, Mirghafourvand M, Mohammad-Alizadeh Charandabi S, *et al.* The effect of ginseng on sexual dysfunction in menopausal women: a double-blind, randomized, controlled trial. *Complement Ther Med.* 2019;45:57-64. doi:10.1016/j.ctim.2019.05.015.

42 Valls-Pedret C, Sala-Vila A, Serra-Mir M, *et al.* Mediterranean diet and age-related cognitive decline: a randomized clinical trial. *JAMA Intern Med.* 2015 Jul;175(7):1094–1103. doi:10.1001/jamainternmed.2015.1668.

43 Xu Y, Zeng L, Zou K, *et al.* Role of dietary factors in the prevention and treatment for depression: an umbrella review of meta-analyses of prospective studies. *Transl Psychiatry.* 2021 Sep 16;11(1):478. doi:10.1038/s41398-021-01590-6. PMID: 34531367.

44 Bonyadi N, Dolatkhah N, Salekzamani Y, *et al.* Effect of berry-based supplements and foods on cognitive function: a systematic review. *Sci Rep.* 2022 Feb 25;12(1):3239. doi:10.1038/s41598-022-07302-4.

45 Puri S, Shaheen M, Grover B. Nutrition and cognitive health: a life course approach. *Front Public Health.* 2023 Mar 27;11:1023907. doi:10.3389/fpubh.2023.1023907. PMID: 37024669; PMCID: PMC10083484.

46 Global Council on Brain Health [Internet]. The real deal on brain health supplements: GCBH recommendations on vitamins, minerals, and other dietary supplements [cited 2025 Feb]. Available from: https://www.aarp.org/content/dam/aarp/health/brain_health/2019/06/gcbh-supplements-report-english.doi.10.26419-2Fpia.00094.001.pdf.

47 Saini RK, Prasad P, Sreedhar RV, *et al.* Omega-3 polyunsaturated fatty acids (PUFAs): emerging plant and microbial sources, oxidative stability, bioavailability, and health benefits—a review. *Antioxidants (Basel).* 2021 Oct 15;10(10):1627. doi:10.3390/antiox10101627.

48 O'Keefe JH Jr, Harris WS. From Inuit to implementation: omega-3 fatty acids come of age. *Mayo Clin Proc.* 2000 Jun;75(6):607-14. doi:10.4065/75.6.607. PMID: 10852422.

49 Yan J, Liu M, Yang D, *et al.* Efficacy and safety of omega-3 fatty acids in the prevention of cardiovascular disease: a systematic review and meta-analysis. *Cardiovasc Drugs Ther.* 2024 Aug;38(4):799-817. doi:10.1007/s10557-022-07379-z.

50 Skulas-Ray AC, Wilson PW, Harris WS, *et al.* Omega-3 fatty acids for the management of hypertriglyceridemia: a science advisory from the American Heart Association. *Circulation.* 2019 Sep 17;140(12):e673-e691. doi:10.1161/CIR.0000000000000709.

51 Lim JC, Caballero Arredondo M, Braakhuis AJ, *et al.* Vitamin C and the lens: new insights into delaying the onset of cataract. *Nutrients.* 2020 Oct 14;12(10):3142. doi:10.3390/nu12103142.

52 Cerullo G, Negro M, Parimbelli M, *et al.* The long history of vitamin C: from prevention of the common cold to potential aid in the treatment of COVID-19. *Front Immunol.* 2020 Oct 28;11:574029. doi:10.3389/fimmu.2020.574029.

53 Wu D, Lewis ED, Pae M, Meydani SN. Nutritional modulation of immune function: analysis of evidence, mechanisms, and clinical relevance. *Front Immunol.* 2018;9:3160. doi:10.3389/fimmu.2018.03160.

54 Stiles LI, Ferrao K, Mehta KJ. Role of zinc in health and disease. *Clin Exp Med.* 2024 Feb 17;24(1):38. doi: 10.1007/s10238-024-01302-6.

55 Chasapis CT, Ntoupa P-SA, Spiliopoulou C, Stefanidou M. Recent aspects of the effects of zinc on human health. *Arch Toxicol.* 2020;94(5):1443-60. doi:10.1007/s00204-020-02702-9.

56 Bhutta ZA, Black RE, Brown KH, *et al.* Prevention of diarrhea and pneumonia by zinc supplementation in children in developing countries: pooled analysis of randomized controlled trials. Zinc Investigators' Collaborative Group. *J Pediatr.* 1999 Dec;135(6):689–97. doi:10.1016/s0022-3476(99)70086-7. PMID: 10586170.

57 Blasiak J, Pawlowska E, Chojnacki J, *et al.* Zinc and autophagy in age-related macular degeneration. *Int J Mol Sci.* 2020 Jul 15;21(14):4994. doi:10.3390/ijms21144994.

58 Ahmad R, Shaju R, Atfi A, *et al.* Zinc and diabetes: a connection between micronutrient and metabolism. *Cells.* 2024 Aug 15;13(16):1359. doi:10.3390/cells13161359.

59 Mozaffar B, Ardavani A, Muzafar H, *et al.* The effectiveness of zinc supplementation in taste disorder treatment: a systematic review and meta-analysis of randomized controlled trials. *Nutr Metab.* 2023 Mar 8;2023:6711071. doi:10.1155/2023/671107.

60 Mousavi SM, Mofrad MD, do Nascimento IJB, *et al.* The effect of zinc supplementation on blood pressure: a systematic review and dose-response meta-analysis of randomized-controlled trials. *Eur J Nutr.* 2020 Aug;59(5):1815–27. doi:10.1007/s00394-020-02204-5.

61 Rychter AM, Hryhorowicz S, Słomski R, *et al.* Antioxidant effects of vitamin E and risk of cardiovascular disease in women with obesity—a narrative review. *Clin Nutr.* 2022 Jul;41(7):1557–65. doi:10.1016/j.clnu.2022.04.032.

62 Yusuf S, Dagenais G, Pogue J, *et al.* Vitamin E supplementation and cardiovascular events in high-risk patients. *N Engl J Med.* 2000 Jan 20;342(3):154-60. doi:10.1056/NEJM200001203420302.

63 Kryscio RJ, Abner EL, Caban-Holt A, *et al.* Association of antioxidant supplement use and dementia in the Prevention of Alzheimer's Disease by Vitamin E and Selenium Trial (PREADViSE). *JAMA Neurol.* 2017;74(5):567-73. doi: 10.1001/jamaneurol.2016.5778.

64 Xin J, Jiang X, Ben S, *et al.* Association between circulating vitamin E and ten common cancers: evidence from large-scale Mendelian randomization analysis and a longitudinal cohort study. *BMC Med.* 2022 May 11;20(1):168. doi:10.1186/s12916-022-02366-5. PMID: 35538486.

65 Jiang H, Yin Y, Wu CR, *et al.* Dietary vitamin and carotenoid intake and risk of age-related cataract. *Am J Clin Nutr.* 2019 Jan 1;109(1):43–54. doi:10.1093/ajcn/nqy270.

66 Hemilä H. Vitamin E administration may decrease the incidence of pneumonia in elderly males. *Clin Interv Aging.* 2016 Oct 3;11:1379–85. doi:10.2147/CIA.S114515.

67 Ibrahim N, Wong SK, Mohamed IN, *et al.* Wound healing properties of selected natural products. *Int J Environ Res Public Health.* 2018 Oct 25;15(11):2360. doi:10.3390/ijerph15112360.

68 Alikamali M, Mohammad-Alizadeh-Charandabi S, Maghalian M, *et al.* The effects of vitamin E on the intensity of primary dysmenorrhea: a systematic review and meta-analysis. *Clin Nutr ESPEN.* 2022 Dec;52:50–9. doi:10.1016/j.clnesp.2022.10.001.

69 Xiong Z, Liu L, Jian Z, *et al.* Vitamin E and multiple health outcomes: an umbrella review of meta-analyses. *Nutrients.* 2023 Jul 25;15(15):3301. doi:10.3390/nu15153301.

70 Hor CP, Fung WY, Ang HA, *et al.* Efficacy of oral mixed tocotrienols in diabetic peripheral neuropathy: a randomized clinical trial. *JAMA Neurol.* 2018;75(4):444-52. doi: 10.1001/jamaneurol.2017.4609.

71 Miller ER 3rd, Pastor-Barriuso R, Dalal D, *et al.* Meta-analysis: high-dosage vitamin E supplementation may increase all-cause mortality. *Ann Intern Med.* 2005 Jan 4;142(1):37–46. doi:10.7326/0003-4819-142-1-200501040-00110.

72 Vivarelli F, Canistro D, Cirillo S, *et al.* Co-carcinogenic effects of vitamin E in prostate. *Sci Rep.* 2019;9:11636. doi:10.1038/s41598-019-48048-0.

73 Méndez López LF, González Llerena JL, Vázquez Rodríguez JA, *et al.* Dietary modulation of the immune system. *Nutrients.* 2024 Dec 18;16(24):4363. doi: 10.3390/nu16244363.

74 Rannem T, Ladefoged K, Hylander E, *et al.* The effect of selenium supplementation on skeletal and cardiac muscle in selenium-depleted patients. *J Parenter Enteral Nutr.* 1995;19(5):351-5. doi:10.1177/0148607195019005351.

75 Jayawardena R, Sooriyaarachchi P, Chourdakis M, *et al.* Enhancing immunity in viral infections, with special emphasis on COVID-19: a review. *Diabetes Metab Syndr.* 2020;14(4):367-82. doi: 10.1016/j.dsx.2020.04.015.

76 Diabetes (India), National Diabetes Obesity and Cholesterol Foundation (NDOC), and Nutrition Expert Group, India. Balanced nutrition is needed in times of COVID-19 epidemic in India: a call for action for all nutritionists and physicians. *Diabetes Metab Syndr*. 2020;14(6):1747-50. doi: 10.1016/j.dsx.2020.08.030.

77 Moghaddam A, Heller R, Sun Q, *et al.* Selenium deficiency is associated with mortality risk from COVID-19. *Nutrients*. 2020;12(7):2098. doi: 10.3390/nu12072098.

78 Tito A, Colantuono A, Pirone L, *et al.* Pomegranate peel extract as an inhibitor of SARS-CoV-2 spike binding to human ACE2 receptor (in vitro): a promising source of novel antiviral drugs. *Front Chem*. 2021 Apr 28;9:638187. doi:10.3389/fchem.2021.638187.

79 Hossain KS, Hossain MG, Moni A, *et al.* Prospects of honey in fighting against COVID-19: pharmacological insights and therapeutic promises. *Heliyon*. 2020 Dec;6(12):e05798. doi:10.1016/j.heliyon.2020.e05798.

80 Koshak AE, Koshak EA, Mobeireek AF, *et al. Nigella sativa* for the treatment of COVID-19: an open-label randomized controlled clinical trial. *Complement Ther Med*. 2021 Sep;61:102769. doi:10.1016/j.ctim.2021.102769.

81 Chong Wang, Ting Wang, Xiao-fei Guo, Duo Li. The associations of fruit and vegetable intake with lung cancer risk in participants with different smoking status: a meta-analysis of prospective cohort studies. *Nutrients*. 2019 Aug 2;11(8):1791. doi: 10.3390/nu11081791.

82 De Cicco P, Catani MV, Gasperi V, *et al.* Nutrition and breast cancer: a literature review on prevention, treatment and recurrence. *Nutrients*. 2019;11(7):1514. doi: 10.3390/nu11071514.

83 Bermejo LM, López-Plaza B, Santurino C, *et al.* Milk and dairy product consumption and bladder cancer risk: a systematic review and meta-analysis of observational studies. *Adv Nutr*. 2019;10(suppl_2):S224-38. doi: 10.1093/advances/nmy119.

84 Applegate C, Rowles J, Ranard K, *et al.* Soy consumption and the risk of prostate cancer: an updated systematic review and meta-analysis. *Nutrients*. 2018;10(1):40. doi: 10.3390/nu10010040.

85 Schwingshackl L, Schwedhelm C, Galbete C, *et al.* Adherence to Mediterranean diet and risk of cancer: an updated systematic review and meta-analysis. *Nutrients*. 2017;9(10):1063. https://doi.org/10.3390/nu9101063.

86 Guasch-Ferré M, Li Y, Willett WC, *et al.* Consumption of olive oil and risk of total and cause-specific mortality among U.S. adults. *J Am Coll Cardiol*. 2022 Jan; 79 (2): 101-12.

87 Aune D, Keum N, Giovannucci E, *et al.* Nut consumption and risk of cardiovascular disease, total cancer, all-cause and cause-specific

mortality: a systematic review and dose-response meta-analysis of prospective studies. *BMC Med*. 2016 Dec 5;14(1):207. doi:10.1186/s12916-016-0730-3.

88 Tomeh A, Hadianamrei R, Zhao Z. A review of curcumin and its derivatives as anticancer agents. *Int J Mol Sci*. 2019;20(5):1033. doi:10.3390/ijms20051033.

89 Ungvari Z, Fekete M, Varga P, *et al*. Association between red and processed meat consumption and colorectal cancer risk: a comprehensive meta-analysis of prospective studies. *Geroscience*. 2025 Apr 10. doi:10.1007/s11357-025-01646-1. Online ahead of print.

90 Fiolet T, Srour B, Sellem L, *et al*. Consumption of ultra-processed foods and cancer risk: results from NutriNet-Santé prospective cohort. *BMJ*. 2018 Feb 14;360:k322. doi:10.1136/bmj.k322.

91 Sargsyan A, Dubasi HB. Milk consumption and prostate cancer: a systematic review. *World J Mens Health*. 2020 Jul 27;39(3):419-28. doi:10.5534/wjmh.200051.

92 Inoue-Choi M, Ramirez Y, O'Connell C, *et al*. Hot beverage intake and oesophageal cancer in the UK Biobank: prospective cohort study. *Br J Cancer*. 2025 Apr;132(7):652–9. doi:10.1038/s41416-025-02953-2. Epub 2025 Feb 19.

93 Debras C, Chazelas E, Srour B, *et al*. Artificial sweeteners and cancer risk: results from the NutriNet-Santé population-based cohort study. *PLoS Med*. 2022 Mar 24;19(3):e1003950. doi:10.1371/journal.pmed.1003950.

94 Shabeer S, Asad S, Jamal A, *et al*. Aflatoxin contamination, its impact and management strategies: an updated review. *Toxins* (*Basel*). 2022 Apr 27;14(5):307. doi:10.3390/toxins14050307.

95 Ravasco P. Nutrition in cancer patients. *J Clin Med*. 2019 Aug 14;8(8):1211. doi:10.3390/jcm8081211.

Chapter 5 Various Foods, Nutrients, Spices and Sweeteners

1 Gopalan C, Rama Sastri BV, Balasubramanian SC. *Nutritive value of Indian foods.* Hyderabad: National Institute of Nutrition, Indian Council of Medical Research; 1989.

2 US Department of Agriculture, Agricultural Research Service. FoodData Central [Internet]. Beltsville (MD): USDA; [cited 2025 Feb]. Available from: https://fdc.nal.usda.gov/fdc-app.html#/food-details/784299/nutrients.

3 US Department of Agriculture, Agricultural Research Service. FoodData Central: Lentils, raw [Internet]. Beltsville (MD): USDA; [cited 2025 Feb]. Available from: https://fdc.nal.usda.gov/fdc-app.html#/food-details/172420/nutrients.

4 Food Standards Australia New Zealand. Australian Food Composition Database [Internet]. Canberra (AU): FSANZ; [cited 2025 Feb]. Available from: https://www.foodstandards.gov.au/.

5 Longvah T, Ananthan R, Bhaskarachary K, Venkaiah K. *Indian food composition tables.* Hyderabad, Telangana: National Institute of Nutrition Indian [Council of Medical Research]; 2017 [cited 2025 Mar]. Available from: https://www.nin.res.in/ebooks/IFCT2017.pdf.

6 Wang C, Ding K, Xie X, *et al.* Soy product consumption and the risk of cancer: a systematic review and meta-analysis of observational studies. *Nutrients.* 2024 Mar 28;16(7):986. doi:10.3390/nu16070986.

7 Kim IS. Current perspectives on the beneficial effects of soybean isoflavones and their metabolites for humans. *Antioxidants (Basel).* 2021 Jun 30;10(7):1064. doi: 10.3390/antiox10071064.

8 Barańska A, Błaszczuk A, Kanadys W, *et al.* Effects of soy protein containing of isoflavones and isoflavones extract on plasma lipid profile in postmenopausal women as a potential prevention factor in cardiovascular diseases: systematic review and meta-analysis of randomized controlled trials. *Nutrients.* 2021 Jul 24;13(8):2531. doi: 10.3390/nu13082531.

9 Franco OH, Chowdhury R, Troup J, *et al.* Use of plant-based therapies and menopausal symptoms: a systematic review and meta-analysis. *JAMA.* 2016 Jun 21;315(23):2554-63. doi: 10.1001/jama.2016.8012.

10 Zuo X, Zhao R, Wu M, *et al.* Soy consumption and the risk of type 2 diabetes and cardiovascular diseases: a systematic review and meta-analysis. *Nutrients.* 2023 Mar 10;15(6):1358. doi: 10.3390/nu15061358.

11 Oldways Whole Grains Council. Definition of a whole grain [Internet]. Boston (MA): Oldways Preservation Trust; [cited 2025 May]. Available from: https://wholegrainscouncil.org/definition-whole-grain.

12 Korczak R. Thinking critically about whole-grain definitions: summary report of an interdisciplinary roundtable discussion at the 2015 Whole Grains Summit. *Am J Clin Nutr.* 2016;104(6):1508-14.

13 Kelly SA, Hartley L, Loveman E, *et al.* Whole grain cereals for the primary or secondary prevention of cardiovascular disease. *Cochrane Database Syst Rev.* 2017;8:CD005051. doi: 10.1002/14651858.CD005051.pub3.

14 Aune D, Giovannucci E, Boffetta P, *et al.* Whole grain consumption and risk of cardiovascular disease, cancer, and all-cause and cause-specific mortality: systematic review and dose-response meta-analysis of prospective studies. *BMJ.* 2016;353:i2716. doi: 10.1136/bmj.i2716.

15 Maki KC, Palacios OM, Koecher K, *et al.* The relationship between whole grain intake and body weight: results of meta-analyses of

observational studies and randomized controlled trials. *Nutrients*. 2019 Jun;11(6):1245. doi: 10.3390/nu11061245.

16 Aloo SO, Ofosu FK, Kilonzi SM, *et al.* Edible plant sprouts: health benefits, trends, and opportunities for novel exploration. *Nutrients*. 2021 Aug 21;13(8):2882. doi: 10.3390/nu13082882.

17 Gold B. What's the difference between whole wheat, whole grain, and multigrain bread? Real Simple. 2025 Feb 28 [cited 2025 Feb]. Available from: https://www.realsimple.com/food-recipes/cooking-tips-techniques/whole-wheat-whole-grain-breads-0.

18 Yusof BN, Talib RA, Karim NA, Kamarudin NA, Arshad F. Glycaemic index of four commercially available breads in Malaysia. *Int J Food Sci Nutr*. 2009 Sep;60(6):487-96. doi: 10.1080/09637480701804268.

19 Najjar AM, Parsons PM, Duncan AM, Robinson LE, Ybarra J, Graham TE. The acute impact of ingestion of breads of varying composition on blood glucose, insulin and incretins following first and second meals. *Br J Nutr*. 2009;101(3):391–8. doi: 10.1017/S0007114508003085.

20 Nowak V, Du J, Charrondiere U. Assessment of the nutritional composition of quinoa (*Chenopodium quinoa Willd.*). *Food Chem*. 2016;193:47-54. doi: 10.1016/j.foodchem.2015.02.111.

21 Misra A, Rastogi K, Joshi S. Whole grains and health: perspective for Asian Indians. *J Assoc Physicians India*. 2009;57:155-62.

22 Priyanka P, Verma S, Singh D. Glycemic index profiling of quinoa (*Chenopodium quinoa Willd*) variety. *J Pharm Res Int*. 2018;21(2):1-5. Article no. JPRI.37915.

23 Mani UV, Prabhu BM, Damle SS. Glycemic index of some commonly consumed foods in Western India. *Asia Pac J Clin Nutr*. 1993;2(3):111-4.

24 Atkinson FS, Foster-Powell K, Brand-Miller JC. International tables of glycemic index and glycemic load values: 2008. *Diabetes Care*. 2008;31(12):2281-3.

25 US Department of Agriculture. USDA food composition databases [cited 2025 Feb]. Available from: https://fdc.nal.usda.gov.

26 Maradini Filho AM, Pirozi MR, Borges JT, *et al.* Quinoa: nutritional, functional, and antinutritional aspects. *Crit Rev Food Sci Nutr*. 2017;57(8):1618-30.

27 Tang Y, Tsao R. Phytochemicals in quinoa and amaranth grains and their antioxidant, anti-inflammatory, and potential health beneficial effects: a review. *Mol Nutr Food Res*. 2017;61(7):1600767. doi: 10.1002/mnfr.201600767.

28 Shobana S, Krishnaswamy K, Sudha V. Finger millet (*Eleusine coracana* L.): a review of its nutritional properties, processing, and plausible health benefits. *Adv Food Nutr Res*. 2013;69:1-39. doi: 10.1016/B978-0-12-410540-9.00001-6.

29 Gulati S, Misra A, Sharma M. Effects of 3 g of soluble fiber from oats on lipid levels of Asian Indians—a randomized controlled, parallel arm study. *Lipids Health Dis*. 2017;16(1):71. doi: 10.1186/s12944-017-0460-3.

30 Li X, Cai X, Ma X. Short- and long-term effects of wholegrain oat intake on weight management and glucolipid metabolism in overweight type-2 diabetics: a randomized control trial. *Nutrients*. 2016;8(9):E549. doi: 10.3390/nu8090549.

31 Smulders MJ, van de Wiel CC, van den Broeck HC. Oats in healthy gluten-free and regular diets: a perspective. *Food Res Int*. 2018;110:3-10. doi: 10.1016/j.foodres.2017.11.031.

32 Rasane P, Jha A, Sabikhi L, *et al*. Nutritional advantages of oats and opportunities for its processing as value added foods—a review. *J Food Sci Technol*. 2013 Jun 25;52(2):662–75. doi:10.1007/s13197-013-1072-1.

33 Foster-Powell K, Holt SH, Brand-Miller JC. International table of glycemic index and glycemic load values: 2002. *Am J Clin Nutr*. 2002;76(1):5-56.

34 Sun Q, Spiegelman D, van Dam RM. White rice, brown rice, and risk of type 2 diabetes in US men and women. *Arch Intern Med*. 2010;170(11):961-9. doi: 10.1001/archinternmed.2010.10.

35 Hamad S, Zafar TA, Sidhu J. Parboiled rice metabolism differs in healthy and diabetic individuals with similar improvement in glycemic response. *Nutrition*. 2018 Mar;47:43-9. doi: 10.1016/j.nut.2017.09.010. Epub 2017 Oct 12.

36 Dujovne CA. Red yeast rice preparations: are they suitable substitutions for statins? *Am J Med*. 2017;130(10):1148-50. doi: 10.1016/j.amjmed.2017.05.013.

37 Murata Y, Hemmi S, Akiya Y, *et al*. Certain red yeast rice supplements in Japan cause acute tubulointerstitial injury. *Kidney Int Rep*. 2024 Sep;9(9):2824–8.

38 Zhang X, Zhao Y, Song Y, *et al*. Effects of *Momordica charantia* L. supplementation on glycemic control and lipid profile in type 2 diabetes mellitus patients: a systematic review and meta-analysis of randomized controlled trials. *Heliyon*. 2024 May 11;10(10):e31126. doi:10.1016/j.heliyon.2024.e31126.

39 Fan M, Kim EK, Choi YJ, *et al*. The role of *Momordica charantia* in resisting obesity. *Int J Environ Res Public Health*. 2019 Sep 4;16(18):3251. doi:10.3390/ijerph16183251.

40 Gong J, Fang K, Dong H, *et al*. Effect of fenugreek on hyperglycaemia and hyperlipidemia in diabetes and prediabetes: a meta-analysis. *J Ethnopharmacol*. 2016 Dec 24;194:260–8. doi:10.1016/j.jep.2016.08.003.

41 Zameer S, Najmi AK, Vohora D, *et al.* A review on therapeutic potentials of *Trigonella foenum-graecum* (fenugreek) and its chemical constituents in neurological disorders: complementary roles to its hypolipidemic, hypoglycemic, and antioxidant potential. *Nutr Neurosci.* 2018 Oct;21(8):539–45. doi:10.1080/1028415X.2017.1327200.

42 Dwitiyanti D, Rachmania RA, Efendi K. In vivo activities and in silico study of jackfruit seeds (*Artocarpus heterophyllus* Lam.) on the reduction of blood sugar levels of gestational diabetes rate induced by streptozotocin. *Open Access Maced J Med Sci.* 2019 Nov 14;7(22):3819-26. doi: 10.3889/oamjms.2019.512. eCollection 2019 Nov 30.

43 Rao AG, Naik KS, Unnikrishnan AG. Efficacy of green jackfruit flour as a medical nutrition therapy replacing rice or wheat in patients with type 2 diabetes mellitus: a randomized, double-blind, placebo-controlled study. *Nutr Diabetes.* 2021 Jun 14;11(1):18. doi: 10.1038/s41387-021-00161-4.

44 Gupta A, Marquess AR, Pandey AK, *et al.* Jackfruit (*Artocarpus heterophyllus* Lam.) in health and disease: a critical review. *Crit Rev Food Sci Nutr.* 2023;63(23):6344-78. doi:10.1080/10408398.2022.2031094. Epub 2022 Feb 10.

45 Gründemann C, Reinhardt JK, Lindequist U. European medicinal mushrooms: do they have potential for modern medicine? - An update. *Phytomedicine.* 2020 Jan;66:153131. doi: 10.1016/j.phymed.2019.153131.

46 Yang Y, Zhu D, Qi R, *et al.* Association between intake of edible mushrooms and algae and the risk of cognitive impairment in Chinese older adults. *Nutrients.* 2024 Feb 25;16(5):637. doi: 10.3390/nu16050637.

47 Jayasuriya WJABN, Wanigatunge CA, Fernando GH, *et al.* Hypoglycaemic activity of culinary *Pleurotus ostreatus* and *P. cystidiosus* mushrooms in healthy volunteers and type 2 diabetic patients on diet control and the possible mechanisms of action. *Phytother Res.* 2015 Feb;29(2):303–9. doi:10.1002/ptr.5255.

48 Mathews JN, Flatt PR, Abdel-Wahab YH, *et al. Asparagus adscendens* (Shweta musali) stimulates insulin secretion, insulin action and inhibits starch digestion. *Br J Nutr.* 2006 Mar;95(3):576–81. doi:10.1079/bjn20051650.

49 Hannan JMA, Ali L, Khaleque J, *et al.* Antihyperglycaemic activity of *Asparagus racemosus* roots is partly mediated by inhibition of carbohydrate digestion and absorption, and enhancement of cellular insulin action. *Br J Nutr.* 2012 May;107(9):1316–23. doi:10.1017/S0007114511004284.

50 Takanari J, Nakahigashi J, Sato A, *et al.* Effect of enzyme-treated asparagus extract (ETAS) on psychological stress in healthy individuals. *J Nutr Sci Vitaminol* (Tokyo). 2016;62(3):198–205. doi:10.3177/jnsv.62.198.

51 Thanakosai W, Phuwapraisirisan P. First identification of α-glucosidase inhibitors from okra (*Abelmoschus esculentus*) seeds. *Nat Prod Commun.* 2013 Aug;8(8):1085–8.

52 Tian ZH, Miao FT, Zhang X, *et al.* Therapeutic effect of okra extract on gestational diabetes mellitus rats induced by streptozotocin. *Asian Pac J Trop Med.* 2015 Dec;8(12):1038–42. doi:10.1016/j.apjtm.2015.11.002.

53 Gemede HF, Haki GD, Beyene F, *et al.* Proximate, mineral, and antinutrient compositions of indigenous okra (*Abelmoschus esculentus*) pod accessions: implications for mineral bioavailability. *Food Sci Nutr.* 2015 Sep 17;4(2):223–33. doi:10.1002/fsn3.282.

54 Kim HJ, Lee KW, Lee HJ. Effect of Nelumbo nucifera rhizome extract on postprandial blood glucose in streptozotocin-induced diabetic rats. *J Food Sci* 2015;80(2); H450-5.

55 Wang Y, Yin J, Nie S, *et al.* Structural characterization and antioxidant activities of polysaccharides from lotus roots. *Carbohydr Polym.* 2016;144:194-204; doi:10.1016/j.carbpol.2016.02.054.

56 Lim SH, Kim YJ, Lee JH, *et al.* Lotus root hot water extract improves lipid metabolism and reduces inflammation in diet-induced obese rats. *Nutr Res Pract.* 2014;8(6);638-45. doi:10.4162/nrp.2014.8.6.638.

57 Hashemian M, Murphy G, Etemadi A, *et al.* Potato consumption and the risk of overall and cause specific mortality in the NIH-AARP study. *PLoS One.* 2019 May 7;14(5):e0216348. doi:10.1371/journal.pone.0216348.

58 Veronese N, Stubbs B, Noale M. Fried potato consumption is associated with elevated mortality: an 8-y longitudinal cohort study. *Am J Clin Nutr.* 2017;106(1):162–7. doi: 10.3945/ajcn.117.154872.

59 Larsson SC, Wolk A. Potato consumption and risk of cardiovascular disease: 2 prospective cohort studies. *Am J Clin Nutr.* 2016;104(5):1245–52.

60 Zhang Z, Venn BJ, Monro J, *et al.* Subjective satiety following meals incorporating rice, pasta and potato. *Nutrients.* 2018 Nov 12;10(11):1739. doi: 10.3390/nu10111739.

61 Su Y, Liu X, Jiang B. Potato intake and the risk of overweight/obesity, hypertension, diabetes, and cardiovascular disease: a systematic review and meta-analysis of observational studies. *Nutr Rev.* 2025 Mar 1;83(3):466–78. doi: 10.1093/nutrit/nuae159.

62 Zhang Y, You D, Lu N, *et al.* Potatoes consumption and risk of type 2 diabetes: a meta-analysis. *Iran J Public Health.* 2018 Nov;47(11):1627–35.

63 Mousavi SM, Gu X, Imamura F, *et al.* Total and specific potato intake and risk of type 2 diabetes: results from three US cohort studies and a substitution meta-analysis of prospective cohorts. *BMJ.* 2025;390:e082121. doi:10.1136/bmj-2024-082121.

64 Henry CJ, Lightowler HJ, Strik CM, *et al.* Glycaemic index values for commercially available potatoes in Great Britain. *Br J Nutr.* 2005;94(6):917–21.

65 Fernandes G, Velangi A, Wolever TM. Glycemic index of potatoes commonly consumed in North America. *J Am Diet Assoc.* 2005;105(4):557–62.

66 Borgi L, Rimm EB, Willett WC. Potato intake and incidence of hypertension: results from three prospective US cohort studies. *BMJ.* 2016;353:i2351. doi: 10.1136/bmj.i2351.

67 Mesias M, Delgado-Andrade C, Holgado F, *et al.* Acrylamide in French fries prepared at primary school canteens. *Food Funct.* 2020;11(2):1489-97. doi:10.1039/c9fo02482d.

68 Shamla L, Nisha P. Acrylamide in deep-fried snacks of India. *Food Addit Contam Part B Surveill.* 2014;7(3):220–5. doi: 10.1080/19393210.2014.894141.

69 Naruszewicz M, Zapolska-Downar D, Kosmider A. Chronic intake of potato chips in humans increases the production of reactive oxygen radicals by leukocytes and increases plasma C-reactive protein: a pilot study. *Am J Clin Nutr.* 2009;89(3):773–7. doi: 10.3945/ajcn.2008.26647.

70 Gurmu F, Hussein S, Laing M. The potential of orange-fleshed sweet potato to prevent vitamin A deficiency in Africa. *Int J Vitam Nutr Res.* 2014;84(1-2):65-78. doi: 10.1024/0300-9831/a000194.

71 Ooi CP, Loke SC. Sweet potato for type 2 diabetes mellitus. *Cochrane Database Syst Rev.* 2013 Sep 3;(9):CD009128. doi: 10.1002/14651858.CD009128.

72 Shih CK, Chen CM, Hsiao TJ. White sweet potato as meal replacement for overweight white-collar workers: a randomized controlled trial. *Nutrients.* 2019 Jan 11;11(1):165. doi: 10.3390/nu11010165.

73 Li N, Wu X, Zhuang W, *et al.* Tomato and lycopene and multiple health outcomes: umbrella review. *Food Chem.* 2021;343:128396. doi:10.1016/j.foodchem.2020.128396.

74 Hurtado-Barroso S, Martínez-Huélamo M, Alverenga JFR, *et al.* Acute effect of a single dose of tomato sofrito on plasmatic inflammatory biomarkers in healthy men. *Nutrients.* 2019 Apr 15;11(4):851. doi: 10.3390/nu11040851.

75 Friedman M. Anticarcinogenic, cardioprotective, and other health benefits of tomato compounds lycopene, α-tomatine, and tomatidine in pure form and in fresh and processed tomatoes. *J Agric Food Chem.* 2013 Oct 9;61(40):9534–50. doi: 10.1021/jf402654e.

76 Grether-Beck S, Marini A, Jaenicke T, *et al.* Molecular evidence that oral supplementation with lycopene or lutein protects human skin against ultraviolet radiation: results from a double-blinded, placebo-controlled, crossover study. *Br J Dermatol.* 2017 May;176(5):1231–40. doi: 10.1111/bjd.15080.

77 Luo J, Ke D, He Q, *et al.* Dietary tomato consumption and the risk of prostate cancer: a meta-analysis. *Front Nutr.* 2021 Feb 25;8:625185. doi: 10.3389/fnut.2021.625185.

78 Cheng HM, Koutsidis G, Lodge JK, *et al.* Tomato and lycopene supplementation and cardiovascular risk factors: a systematic review and meta-analysis. *Atherosclerosis.* 2017 Mar;257:100–8. doi: 10.1016/j.atherosclerosis.2017.01.009.

79 Chen D, Huang C, Chen Z. A review for the pharmacological effect of lycopene in central nervous system disorders. *Biomed Pharmacother.* 2019 Mar;111:791-801. doi: 10.1016/j.biopha.2018.12.151. Epub 2019 Jan 4.

80 Mazidi M, Katsiki N, George ES, *et al.* Tomato and lycopene consumption is inversely associated with total and cause-specific mortality: a population-based cohort study, on behalf of the International Lipid Expert Panel (ILEP). *Br J Nutr.* 2020 Dec 28;124(12):1303-1310. doi: 10.1017/S0007114519002150. Epub 2019 Aug 22.

81 Huang J, Weinstein SJ, Yu K, *et al.* Serum beta carotene and overall and cause-specific mortality. *Circ Res.* 2018 Dec 7;123(12):1339-49. doi: 10.1161/CIRCRESAHA.118.313409.

82 Middha P, Weinstein SJ, Männistö S, *et al.* β-Carotene supplementation and lung cancer incidence in the Alpha-Tocopherol, Beta-Carotene Cancer Prevention Study: the role of tar and nicotine. *Nicotine Tob Res.* 2019;21(8):1045-50. doi: 10.1093/ntr/nty115.

83 Kordiak J, Bielec F, Jabłoński S, *et al.* Role of beta-carotene in lung cancer primary chemoprevention: a systematic review with meta-analysis and meta-regression. *Nutrients.* 2022 Mar 24;14(7):1361. doi: 10.3390/nu14071361.

84 Omenn GS, Goodman GE, Thornquist MD, *et al.* Effects of a combination of beta carotene and vitamin A on lung cancer and cardiovascular disease. *N Engl J Med.* 1996 May 2;334(18):1150-5. doi: 10.1056/NEJM199605023341802.

85 Jiang H, Yin Y, Wu CR, *et al.* Dietary vitamin and carotenoid intake and risk of age-related cataract. *Am J Clin Nutr.* 2019 Jan 1;109(1):43-54. doi: 10.1093/ajcn/nqy270. PMID: 30624584.

86 Di Pierro E, Granata F. Nutrients and porphyria: an intriguing crosstalk. *Int J Mol Sci.* 2020 May 14;21(10):3462. doi: 10.3390/ijms21103462. PMID: 32422947.
87 Shukla K, Narain JP, Puri P, *et al.* Glycaemic response to maize, bajra and barley. *Indian J Physiol Pharmacol.* 1991 Oct;35(4):249-54.
88 Soong YY, Quek RY, Henry CJ, *et al.* Glycemic potency of muffins made with wheat, rice, corn, oat and barley flours: a comparative study between in vivo and in vitro. *Eur J Nutr.* 2015;54(8):1281-5. doi: 10.1007/s00394-014-0806-9.
89 Armah CN, Derdemezis C, Traka MH, *et al.* Diet rich in high glucoraphanin broccoli reduces plasma LDL cholesterol: evidence from randomised controlled trials. *Mol Nutr Food Res.* 2015;59(5):918-26. doi: 10.1002/mnfr.201400863.
90 Bessler H, Djaldetti M, *et al.* Broccoli and human health: immunomodulatory effect of sulforaphane in a model of colon cancer. *Int J Food Sci Nutr.* 2018;69(8):946-53. doi: 10.1080/09637486.2018.1439901.
91 Chen JG, Johnson J, Egner P, *et al.* Dose-dependent detoxication of the airborne pollutant benzene in a randomized trial of broccoli sprout beverage in Qidong, China. *Am J Clin Nutr.* 2019;110(3):675-84. doi: 10.1093/ajcn/nqz122.
92 Kikuchi M, Ushida Y, Shiozawa H, *et al.* Sulforaphane-rich broccoli sprout extract improves hepatic abnormalities in male subjects. *World J Gastroenterol.* 2015;21(43):12457-67. doi: 10.3748/wjg.v21.i43.12457.
93 Dwibedi C, Axelsson AS, Abrahamsson B, *et al.* Effect of broccoli sprout extract and baseline gut microbiota on fasting blood glucose in prediabetes: a randomized, placebo-controlled trial. *Nat Microbiol.* 2025 Feb 10. doi: 10.1038/s41564-025-01932-w.
94 Liu AH, Bondonno CP, Croft KD, *et al.* Effects of a nitrate-rich meal on arterial stiffness and blood pressure in healthy volunteers. *Nitric Oxide.* 2013;35:123-30. doi: 10.1016/j.niox.2013.10.001.
95 Moser B, Szekeres T, Bieglmayer C, *et al.* Impact of spinach consumption on DNA stability in peripheral lymphocytes and on biochemical blood parameters: results of a human intervention trial. *Eur J Nutr.* 2011;50(7):587-94. doi: 10.1007/s00394-011-0167-6.
96 Wen J, Syed B, Abed I, *et al.* Improved effect of spinach extract on physical performance: a systematic review of randomized controlled trials. *Cureus.* 2025;17(1):e77840. doi: 10.7759/cureus.77840.
97 Ganesan K, Xu B, *et al.* Polyphenol-rich dry common bean (*P. vulgaris L.*) and their health benefits. *Int J Mol Sci.* 2017;18(11):E2331. doi: 10.3390/ijms18112331.

98 Winham DM, Hutchins AM, Thompson SV, *et al.* Glycaemic response to black beans and chickpeas as part of a rice meal: a randomized cross-over trial. *Nutrients*. 2017;9(10):E1095. doi: 10.3390/nu9101095.

99 Haas JD, Luna SV, Lung'aho MG, *et al.* Consuming iron biofortified beans increases iron status in Rwandan women after 128 days in a randomized controlled feeding trial. *J Nutr.* 2016;146(8):1586-92. doi: 10.3945/jn.115.224741.

100 Doma KM, Dolinar KF, Ramdath DD, *et al.* Canned beans decrease serum total and LDL cholesterol in adults with elevated LDL cholesterol in a 4-week multicenter, randomized, crossover study. *J Nutr.* 2021;151(12):3701-9. doi: 10.1093/jn/nxab323.

101 Trinidad PT, Mallillin AC, Loyola AS, *et al.* The potential health benefits of legumes as a good source of dietary fibre. *Br J Nutr.* 2010;103(4):569-74. doi: 10.1017/S0007114509992157.

102 Saadh MJ, Kariem M, Shukla M, *et al.* Effects of aged garlic extract on blood pressure in hypertensive patients: a systematic review and meta-analysis of randomized controlled trials. *Prostaglandins Other Lipid Mediat.* 2024 Dec;175:106914. doi: 10.1016/j.prostaglandins.2024.106914.

103 Darooghegi Mofrad M, Milajerdi A, Koohdani F, *et al.* Garlic supplementation reduces circulating C-reactive protein, tumor necrosis factor, and interleukin-6 in adults: a systematic review and meta-analysis of randomized controlled trials. *J Nutr.* 2019 Apr 1;149(4):605–18. doi: 10.1093/jn/nxy310.

104 Shabani E, Sayemiri K, Mohammadpour M. The effect of garlic on lipid profile and glucose parameters in diabetic patients: a systematic review and meta-analysis. *Prim Care Diabetes.* 2019 Feb;13(1):28–42. doi: 10.1016/j.pcd.2018.07.007.

105 Guercio V, Turati F, La Vecchia C, *et al.* Allium vegetables and upper aerodigestive tract cancers: a meta-analysis of observational studies. *Mol Nutr Food Res.* 2016 Jan;60(1):212–22. doi: 10.1002/mnfr.201500587.

106 Hosseinzadeh-Attar MJ, Alipoor E, Dehghani S, Salimzadeh A. Increased efficacy of a garlic supplement on knee osteoarthritis symptoms in patients with obesity. *J Herb Med.* 2020 Dec;24:100392. doi: 10.1016/j.hermed.2020.100392.

107 Hiyasat B, Sabha D, Grotzinger K, *et al.* Antiplatelet activity of *Allium ursinum* and *Allium sativum*. *Pharmacology.* 2009;83(4):197–204. doi: 10.1159/000196811.

108 Hirsch GE, Viecili PRN, de Almeida AS, *et al.* Natural products with antiplatelet action. *Curr Pharm Des.* 2017;23(8):1228–46. doi: 10.2174/1381612823666161123151611.

109 Kehar S, Bhatt SP, Pandey RM, *et al.* Glycaemic responses to three mango varieties in type 2 diabetes and non-diabetic subjects: a pilot crossover study using OTT and CGM. *Eur J Clin Nutr.* Accepted for publication, 2025.

110 Kehar S, Sharma S, Bhardwaj S, *et al.* Effect of daily consumption of mango (*Mangifera indica*) on glycemia, insulin resistance and anthropometry in individuals with type 2 diabetes: a randomized controlled trial. *J Diabetes Metab Disord.* 2025 Aug 6. Available from: https://pubmed.ncbi.nlm.nih.gov/40761695/.

111 Chandran R, Parimelazhagan T, Shanmugam S, *et al.* Antidiabetic activity of *Syzygium calophyllifolium* in Streptozotocin-Nicotinamide induced Type-2 diabetic rats. *Biomed Pharmacother.* 2016;82:547-54. doi:10.1016/j.biopha.2016.05.036.

112 Teixeira CC, Weinert LS, Barbosa DC, *et al.* *Syzygium cumini* (L.) Skeels in the treatment of type 2 diabetes: results of a randomized, double-blind, double-dummy, controlled trial. *Diabetes Care.* 2004;27(12):3019-20. doi:10.2337/diacare.27.12.3019-a.

113 Liu F, Ma H, Wang G, *et al.* Phenolics from *Eugenia jambolana* seeds with advanced glycation end product formation and alpha-glucosidase inhibitory activities. *Food Funct.* 2018;9(8):4246-54. doi:10.1039/c8fo00583d.

114 Rasheed S, Tahir M, Sami W, *et al.* Histological effects of *Eugenia jambolana* seed extract on liver of adult albino rats. *J Ayub Med Coll Abbottabad.* 2009;21(1):148-51.

115 Schell J, Scofield RH, Barrett JR, Kurien BT, Betts N, Lyons TJ, *et al.* Strawberries improve pain and inflammation in obese adults with radiographic evidence of knee osteoarthritis. *Nutrients.* 2017 Aug 28;9(9):949. doi: 10.3390/nu9090949.

116 Kursvietiene L, Staneviciene I, Mongirdiene A, Bernatoniene J. Multiplicity of effects and health benefits of resveratrol. *Medicina.* 2016;52(3):148-55.

117 Davicco MJ, Wittrant Y, Coxam V. Berries, their micronutrients and bone health. *Curr Opin Clin Nutr Metab Care.* 2016;19(6):453-7. doi:10.1097/MCO.0000000000000324. PMID: 27583710.

118 Kalt W, Cassidy A, Howard LR, *et al.* Recent research on the health benefits of blueberries and their anthocyanins. *Adv Nutr.* 2020;11(2):224-36. doi: 10.1093/advances/nmz065.

119 Johnson SA, Figueroa A, Navaei N, *et al.* Daily blueberry consumption improves blood pressure and arterial stiffness in postmenopausal women with pre- and stage-1 hypertension: a randomized, double-blind, placebo-controlled clinical trial. *J Acad Nutr Diet.* 2015;115(3):369-77.

120 Miller K, Feucht W, Schmid M, *et al.* Bioactive compounds of strawberry and blueberry and their potential health effects based on human intervention studies: a brief overview. *Nutrients.* 2019;11(7):E1510. doi: 10.3390/nu11071510.

121 Curtis PJ, Berends L, van der Velpen V, *et al.* Blueberry anthocyanin intake attenuates the postprandial cardiometabolic effect of an energy-dense food challenge: results from a double-blind, randomized controlled trial in metabolic syndrome participants. *Clin Nutr.* 2022;41(1):165-76. doi: 10.1016/j.clnu.2021.11.030.

122 Gao X, Cassidy A, Schwarzschild MA, Rimm EB, Ascherio A. Habitual intake of dietary flavonoids and risk of Parkinson disease. *Neurology.* 2012;78:1138–45.

123 Blum JE, Gheller BJ, Hwang S, *et al.* Consumption of a blueberry-enriched diet by women for 6 weeks alters determinants of human muscle progenitor cell function. *J Nutr.* 2020 Sep 1;150(9):2412-8. doi: 10.1093/jn/nxaa190.

124 Upadya H, Prabhu S, Prasad A, *et al.* A randomized, double-blind, placebo-controlled, multicentre clinical trial to assess the efficacy and safety of *Emblica officinalis* extract in patients with dyslipidemia. *BMC Complement Altern Med.* 2019;19(1):27. doi: 10.1186/s12906-019-2430-y.

125 Fatima N, Hafizur RM, Hameed A, *et al.* Ellagic acid in *Emblica officinalis* exerts anti-diabetic activity through the action on β-cells of pancreas. *Eur J Nutr.* 2017 Mar;56(2):591-601. doi: 10.1007/s00394-015-1103-y.

126 Amor V, Amor C, Giron MD, *et al.* Ellagic acid as a tool to limit the diabetes burden: updated evidence. *Antioxidants* (*Basel*). 2020;9(12):1226. doi: 10.3390/antiox9121226.

127 Setayesh L, Clark CC, Pourbagher-Shahri AM, *et al.* The impact of *Emblica officinalis* (Amla) on lipid profile, glucose, and C-reactive protein: a systematic review and meta-analysis of randomized controlled trials. *Diabetes Metab Syndr.* 2023;17(3):102729. doi: 10.1016/j.dsx.2023.102729.

128 Usharani V, Fatima N, Muralidhar N, *et al.* Effects of *Phyllanthus emblica* extract on endothelial dysfunction and biomarkers of oxidative stress in patients with type 2 diabetes mellitus: a randomized, double-blind, controlled study. *Diabetes Metab Syndr Obes.* 2013;6:275-84. doi: 10.2147/DMSO.S46341.

129 Tiwari V, Kuhad A, Chopra K. *Emblica officinalis* corrects functional, biochemical and molecular deficits in experimental diabetic neuropathy by targeting the oxido-nitrosative stress mediated inflammatory cascade. *Phytother Res.* 2011 Oct;25(10):1527-36. doi: 10.1002/ptr.3440.

130 Suryanarayana P, Saraswat M, Petrash JM, *et al. Emblica officinalis* and its enriched tannoids delay streptozotocin-induced diabetic cataract in rats. *Mol Vis.* 2007 Jul 24;13:1291-7.

131 Dreher ML, Davenport AJ. Hass avocado composition and potential health effects. *Crit Rev Food Sci Nutr.* 2013;53(7):738–50. doi:10.1080/10408398.2011.556759.

132 Li Z, Wong A, Henning SM, *et al.* Hass avocado modulates postprandial vascular reactivity and postprandial inflammatory responses to a hamburger meal in healthy volunteers. *Food Funct.* 2013 Feb 26;4(3):384–91. doi:10.1039/c2fo30226h.

133 James-Martin G, Brooker PG, Hendrie GA, *et al.* Avocado consumption and cardiometabolic health: a systematic review and meta-analysis. *J Acad Nutr Diet.* 2024 Feb;124(2):233–248.e4. doi:10.1016/j.jand.2022.12.008.

134 Matthan NR, Lovato L, Petersen KS, *et al.* Effect of daily avocado consumption for 6 mo compared with habitual diet on red blood cell fatty acid profiles and association with cardiometabolic risk factors in individuals with abdominal obesity: a randomized trial. *Am J Clin Nutr.* 2024 Oct;120(4):794–803. doi:10.1016/j.ajcnut.2024.08.002.

135 Wien M, Haddad E, Oda K, *et al.* A randomized 3×3 crossover study to evaluate the effect of Hass avocado intake on post-ingestive satiety, glucose and insulin levels, and subsequent energy intake in overweight adults. *Nutr J.* 2013 Nov 27;12:155. doi:10.1186/1475-2891-12-155.

136 Scott TM, Rasmussen HM, Chen O, *et al.* Avocado consumption increases macular pigment density in older adults: a randomized, controlled trial. *Nutrients.* 2017 Aug 23;9(9):919. doi:10.3390/nu9090919.

137 Edwards CG, Walk AM, Thompson SV, *et al.* Effects of 12-week avocado consumption on cognitive function among adults with overweight and obesity. *Int J Psychophysiol.* 2020 Feb;148:13–24. doi:10.1016/j.ijpsycho.2019.12.006.

138 Kotha R, Luthria D. Curcumin: biological, pharmaceutical, nutraceutical, and analytical aspects. *Molecules.* 2019;24(16):2930. doi:10.3390/molecules24162930.

139 Ono K, Hasegawa K, Naiki H, *et al.* Curcumin has potent anti-amyloidogenic effects for Alzheimer's beta-amyloid fibrils in vitro. *J Neurosci Res.* 2004;75(6):742–50.

140 Rodrigues FC, Anil Kumar NV, Thakur G. Developments in the anticancer activity of structurally modified curcumin: an up-to-date review. *Eur J Med Chem.* 2019 Sep 1;177:76–104. doi:10.1016/j.ejmech.2019.04.058.

141 Giordano A, Tommonaro G. Curcumin and cancer. *Nutrients.* 2019;11(10):2376. doi:10.3390/nu11102376.

142 Kumari A, Raina N, Wahi A, *et al.* Wound-healing effects of curcumin and its nanoformulations: a comprehensive review. *Pharmaceutics.* 2022 Oct 25;14(11):2288. doi:10.3390/pharmaceutics14112288.

143 Yaikwawong M, Jansarikit L, Jirawatnotai S, *et al.* Curcumin extract improves beta cell functions in obese patients with type 2 diabetes: a randomized controlled trial. *Nutr J.* 2024 Oct 1;23(1):119. doi:10.1186/s12937-024-01022-3.

144 Motlagh Asghari K, Saleh P, Salekzamani Y, *et al.* The effect of curcumin and high-content eicosapentaenoic acid supplementations in type 2 diabetes mellitus patients: a double-blinded randomized clinical trial. *Nutr Diabetes.* 2024 Apr 8;14(1):14. doi:10.1038/s41387-024-00274-6.

145 Unhapipatpong C, Phuseerit W, Wongviriyawong T, *et al.* The effect of curcumin supplementation on weight loss and anthropometric indices: an umbrella review and updated meta-analyses of randomized controlled trials. *Am J Clin Nutr.* 2023;117(5):1005–16. doi:10.1016/j.ajcnut.2023.03.006.

146 Yaikwawong M, Jansarikit L, Jirawatnotai S, *et al.* Curcumin reduces depression in obese patients with type 2 diabetes: a randomized controlled trial. *Nutrients.* 2024 Jul 25;16(15):2414. doi:10.3390/nu16152414.

147 He Y, Chen X, Li Y, *et al.* Curcumin supplementation alleviates hepatic fat content associated with modulation of gut microbiota-dependent bile acid metabolism in patients with nonalcoholic simple fatty liver disease: a randomized controlled trial. *Am J Clin Nutr.* 2024 Jul;120(1):66-79.

148 Tanabe Y, Kondo E, Sagayama H, *et al.* Impact of curcumin supplementation on exercise performance and muscle damage after a soccer match: a double-blind placebo-controlled cross-over study. *Eur J Appl Physiol.* 2024 Jul;124(7):2161–70. doi:10.1007/s00421-024-05429-y.

149 Yallapu MM, Jaggi M, Chauhan SC. Therapeutic applications of curcumin nanoformulations. *AAPS J.* 2015;17(6):1341–56.

150 Committee on Toxicity. First draft statement on the potential risk to human health of turmeric and curcumin [Internet]. London: Food Standards Agency. Available from: https://cot.food.gov.uk.

151 Gupta Jain S, Puri S, Misra A, *et al.* Effect of oral cinnamon intervention on metabolic profile and body composition of Asian Indians with metabolic syndrome: a randomized double-blind control trial. *Lipids Health Dis.* 2017;16(1):113. doi:10.1186/s12944-017-0504-8. (Paper from our group).

152 Santos HO, da Silva GAR, *et al.* To what extent does cinnamon administration improve the glycemic and lipid profiles? *Clin Nutr ESPEN.* 2018;27:1-9. doi:10.1016/j.clnesp.2018.07.011.

153 Soares AP da C, de Faria NC, Graciano GF, *et al.* Cinnamon infusion reduces satiety and increases energy intake: a randomized crossover trial. *Ann Nutr Metab.* 2022;78(5):265-72. doi:10.1159/000525949.

154 Momtaz S, Hassani S, Khan F, *et al.* Cinnamon, a promising prospect towards Alzheimer's disease. *Pharmacol Res.* 2018;130:241-58. doi:10.1016/j.phrs.2017.12.011.

155 Refaei M, Karami Z, Kazemi F, *et al.* Cinnamon potential in alleviating early postmenopause symptoms: a randomized clinical trial. *Menopause.* 2024;31(12):1078-84. doi:10.1097/GME.0000000000002444.

156 Bitok E, Sabaté J. Nuts and cardiovascular disease. *Prog Cardiovasc Dis.* 2018;61(1):33-37. doi:10.1016/j.pcad.2018.05.003.

157 Nishi S, Kendall CWC, Gascoyne AM, *et al.* Nuts in the prevention and management of type 2 diabetes. *Nutrients.* 2023;15(4):878. doi:10.3390/nu15040878.

158 Trumbo PR, Ard J, Bellisle F, *et al.* Perspective: current scientific evidence and research strategies in the role of almonds in cardiometabolic health. *Curr Dev Nutr.* 2025;9(1):104516. doi:10.1016/j.cdnut.2024.104516.

159 Gulati S, Misra A, Pandey RM, *et al.* Effects of pistachio nuts on body composition, metabolic, inflammatory and oxidative stress parameters in Asian Indians with metabolic syndrome: a 24-wk, randomized control trial. *Nutrition.* 2014;30(2):192-7. doi:10.1016/j.nut.2013.08.005.

160 Gulati S, Misra A, Pandey RM. Effect of almond supplementation on glycemia and cardiovascular risk factors in Asian Indians in North India with type 2 diabetes mellitus: a 24-week study. *Metab Syndr Relat Disord.* 2017;15(2):98-105. doi:10.1089/met.2016.0066.

161 Gulati S, Misra A, Tiwari R, *et al.* Premeal almond load decreases postprandial glycaemia, adiposity and reversed prediabetes to normoglycemia: a randomized controlled trial. *Clin Nutr ESPEN.* 2023;54:12-22. doi:10.1016/j.clnesp.2022.12.028.

162 Gulati S, Misra A, Tiwari R, *et al.* Beneficial effects of premeal almond load on glucose profile on oral glucose tolerance and continuous glucose monitoring: randomized crossover trials in Asian Indians with prediabetes. *Eur J Clin Nutr.* 2023;77(5):586-95. doi:10.1038/s41430-023-01263-1.

163 Klimova B, Kuca K, Valis M, *et al.* Role of nut consumption in the management of cognitive decline—a mini-review. *Curr Alzheimer Res.* 2018;15(9):877-882. doi:10.2174/1567205015666180202100721.

164 Chen GC, Zhang R, Martínez-González MA, *et al.* Nut consumption in relation to all-cause and cause-specific mortality: a meta-analysis 18 prospective studies. *Food Funct.* 2017;8(11):3893-3905. doi:10.1039/c7fo00915a.

165 Salas-Huetos A, Muralidharan J, Galiè S, *et al.* Effect of nut consumption on erectile and sexual function in healthy males: a secondary outcome analysis of the FERTINUTS randomized controlled trial. *Nutrients.* 2019;11(6):E1372. doi:10.3390/nu11061372.

166 Hernández-Alonso P, Camacho-Barcia L, Bulló M, *et al.* Nuts and dried fruits: an update of their beneficial effects on type 2 diabetes. *Nutrients.* 2017;9(7):E673. doi:10.3390/nu9070673.

167 Anderson JW, Waters AR. Raisin consumption by humans: effects on glycemia and insulinemia and cardiovascular risk factors. *J Food Sci.* 2013;78:A11-A17.

168 Kim Y, Hertzler SR, Byrne HK, *et al.* Raisins are a low to moderate glycaemic index food with correspondingly low insulin index. *Nutr Res.* 2008;28(5):304-308.

169 Bajaj M, Misra A. Effect of dates on blood glucose and other metabolic variables: a narrative review. *Diabetes Metab Syndr.* 2023 [cited 2025 Mar 2].

170 Gonzales-Malca JA, Tirado-Kulieva VA, Abanto-López MS, *et al.* Worldwide research on the health effects of bovine milk containing A1 and A2 β-casein: unraveling the current scenario and future trends through bibliometrics and text mining. *Curr Res Food Sci.* 2023 Sep 23;7:100602. doi: 10.1016/j.crfs.2023.100602.

171 Erlich MN, Ghidanac D, Blanco Mejia S, *et al.* A systematic review and meta-analysis of randomized trials of substituting soymilk for cow's milk and intermediate cardiometabolic outcomes: understanding the impact of dairy alternatives in the transition to plant-based diets on cardiometabolic health. *BMC Med.* 2024 Aug 22;22(1):336. doi: 10.1186/s12916-024-03524-7.

172 Feskanich D, Meyer HE, Fung TT, *et al.* Milk and other dairy foods and risk of hip fracture in men and women. *Osteoporos Int.* 2018 Feb;29(2):385-396. doi: 10.1007/s00198-017-4285-8.

173 Ong AM, Kang K, Weiler HA, *et al.* Fermented milk products and bone health in postmenopausal women: a systematic review of randomized controlled trials, prospective cohorts, and case-control studies. *Adv Nutr.* 2020;11(2):251-265. doi: 10.1093/advances/nmz108.

174 Willett WC, Ludwig DS. Milk and health. *N Engl J Med.* 2020;382(7):644-654. doi: 10.1056/NEJMra1903547.

175 Vanderhout SM, Aglipay M, Torabi N, *et al.* Whole milk compared with reduced-fat milk and childhood overweight: a systematic review and meta-analysis. *Am J Clin Nutr.* 2020 Feb 1;111(2):266-79. doi: 10.1093/ajcn/nqz276. PMID: 31851302.

176 Eales J, Lenoir-Wijnkoop I, King S, *et al.* Is consuming yoghurt associated with weight management outcomes? Results from a

systematic review. *Int J Obes (Lond)*. 2016 May;40(5):731-46. doi: 10.1038/ijo.2015.202. Epub 2015 Oct 7. PMID: 26443336.

177 Giosuè A, Calabrese I, Vitale M, *et al.* Consumption of dairy foods and cardiovascular disease: a systematic review. *Nutrients*. 2022 Feb 16;14(4):831. doi: 10.3390/nu14040831. PMID: 35215479.

178 Zhang M, Dong X, Huang Z, *et al.* Cheese consumption and multiple health outcomes: an umbrella review and updated meta-analysis of prospective studies. *Adv Nutr.* 2023 Sep;14(5):1170-1186. doi: 10.1016/j.advnut.2023.06.007. Epub 2023 Jun 15. PMID: 37328108.

179 de Goede J, Soedamah-Muthu SS, Pan A, *et al.* Dairy consumption and risk of stroke: a systematic review and updated dose-response meta-analysis of prospective cohort studies. *J Am Heart Assoc.* 2016;5(5):e002787. doi: 10.1161/JAHA.115.002787.

180 Lampousi AM, Carlsson S, Löfvenborg JE. Dietary factors and risk of islet autoimmunity and type 1 diabetes: a systematic review and meta-analysis. *EBioMedicine*. 2021 Oct:72:103633. doi: 10.1016/j.ebiom.2021.103633. Epub 2021 Oct 14. PMID: 34656932.

181 Tanpowpong P, Aekplakorn W, Chariyalertsak S, *et al.* Higher milk consumption is associated with a lower risk of diabetes mellitus: a case-control study. *PLoS One*. 2023 Aug 16;18(8):e0289762. doi: 10.1371/journal.pone.0289762. eCollection 2023. PMID: 37585412.

182 Scialo TE, Pace CM, Abrams DI. The dairy and cancer controversy: milking the evidence. *Curr Oncol Rep*. 2024 Mar;26(3):191-199. doi: 10.1007/s11912-024-01496-8. Epub 2024 Jan 30. PMID: 38289521.

183 Misselwitz B, Butter M, Verbeke K, *et al.* Update on lactose malabsorption and intolerance: pathogenesis, diagnosis and clinical management. *Gut*. 2019 Nov;68(11):2080-91. doi: 10.1136/gutjnl-2019-318404. Epub 2019 Aug 19. PMID: 31427404.

184 Yoganandi J, Mehta BM, Wadhwani KN. Evaluation and comparison of camel milk with cow milk and buffalo milk for gross composition. *J Camel Pract Res*. 2014;21(2):259-265. doi: 10.5958/2277-8934.2014.00046.0.

185 Kapadiya DB, Prajapati DB, Jain AK, *et al.* Comparison of Surti goat milk with cow and buffalo milk for gross composition, nitrogen distribution, and selected minerals content. *Vet World*. 2016;9(7):710-716.

186 Mohapatra A, Shinde AK, Singh R. Sheep milk: a pertinent functional food. *Small Rumin Res*. 2019;181:6-11.

187 Nikkhah A. Science of camel and yak milks: human nutrition and health perspectives. *Food Nutr Sci*. 2011;2(6):667-673.

188 Nikkhah A. Equidae, camel, and yak milks as functional foods: a review. *J Nutr Food Sci*. 2011;1:116.

189 Singh R, Mal G, Kumar D, *et al.* Camel milk: an important natural adjuvant. *Agric Res.* 2017;6:327-340.

190 US Department of Agriculture. Food Data Central: milk, sheep, fluid [Internet]. 2019 [cited 2025 Mar 3]. Available from: https://fdc.nal.usda.gov/fdc-app.html#/food-details/781103/nutrients.

191 US Department of Agriculture. FoodData Central: milk, goat, fluid, with added vitamin D [Internet]. 2019 [cited 2025 Mar 3]. Available from: https://fdc.nal.usda.gov/fdc-app.html#/food-details/172446/nutrients.

192 US Department of Agriculture. FoodData Central: milk, whole, 3.25% milkfat, with added vitamin D. 2019 [cited 2025 Mar 3]. Available from: https://fdc.nal.usda.gov/fdc-app.html#/food-details/174832/nutrients.

193 Skeaff CM, Williscroft K, Mann J. Replacing cows' with sheep's dairy fat lowers plasma cholesterol concentration in participants consuming dairy fat-rich diets. *Eur J Clin Nutr.* 2004 Feb;58(2):250-7. doi: 10.1038/sj.ejcn.1601774. PMID: 14749744.

194 Rafiq S, Huma N, Pasha I, *et al.* Chemical composition, nitrogen fractions and amino acids profile of milk from different animal species. *Asian-Australas J Anim Sci.* 2016;29(7):1022-1028.

195 Shamsia SM. Nutritional and therapeutic properties of camel and human milks. *Int J Genet Mol Biol.* 2009;1(2):52-58.

196 Chen Y, Feng R, Yang X, *et al.* Yogurt improves insulin resistance and liver fat in obese women with non-alcoholic fatty liver disease and metabolic syndrome: a randomized controlled trial. *Am J Clin Nutr.* 2019;109(6):1611-19. doi: 10.1093/ajcn/nqy358.

197 Salas-Salvadó J, Guasch-Ferré M, Díaz-López A, *et al.* Yogurt and diabetes: overview of recent observational studies. *J Nutr.* 2017;147(7):1452S-1461S. doi: 10.3945/jn.117.248229.

198 FDA announces qualified health claim for yogurt and reduced risk of type 2 diabetes. Food & Drug Law Institute. 2024 Mar 1 [cited 2025 Mar 3]. Available from: https://www.fdli.org/2024/05/fda-announces-qualified-health-claim-for-yogurt-and-reduced-risk-of-type-2-diabetes/.

199 Chen GC, Wang Y, Tong X, *et al.* Cheese consumption and risk of cardiovascular disease: a meta-analysis of prospective studies. *Eur J Nutr.* 2017;56(8):2565-75. doi: 10.1007/s00394-016-1292-z.

200 Yuan M, Hu FB, Li Y, *et al.* Types of dairy foods and risk of fragility fracture in the prospective Nurses' Health Study cohort. *Am J Clin Nutr.* 2023 Dec;118(6):1172-81. doi: 10.1016/j.ajcnut.2023.09.015.

201 Leyh SM, Willingham BD, Baur DA, *et al.* Pre-sleep protein in casein supplement or whole-food form has no impact on resting energy

expenditure or hunger in women. *Br J Nutr*. 2018;120(9):988-94. doi: 10.1017/S0007114518002416.

202 Marsset-Baglieri A, Fromentin G, Airinei G, *et al*. The satiating effects of eggs or cottage cheese are similar in healthy subjects despite differences in postprandial kinetics. *Appetite*. 2015;90:136-43. doi: 10.1016/j.appet.2015.03.010.

203 Mittal J. Should we count dietary cholesterol in dairy products? A perspective from India and South Asia. *Diabetes Metab Syndr*. 2020 Mar-Apr;14(2):117. doi: 10.1016/j.dsx.2020.01.013.

204 Misra A. Dietary cholesterol advisory from American Heart Association: implications for India and other developing countries. *Diabetes Metab Syndr*. 2020;14(2):107-8. doi: 10.1016/j.dsx.2020.01.005.

205 Misra A, Sharma R, Gulati S, *et al*. Consensus dietary guidelines for healthy living and prevention of obesity, the metabolic syndrome, diabetes, and related disorders in Asian Indians. *Diabetes Technol Ther*. 2011;13(6):683-94. doi: 10.1089/dia.2010.0198.

206 Réhault-Godbert S, Guyot N, Nys Y, *et al*. The golden egg: nutritional value, bioactivities, and emerging benefits for human health. Nutrients. 2019;11(3):E684. doi: 10.3390/nu11030684.

207 Carson JAS, Lichtenstein AH, Anderson CAM, *et al*. Dietary cholesterol and cardiovascular risk: a science advisory from the American Heart Association. *Circulation*. 2020 Jan 21;141(3):e39-e53. doi: 10.1161/CIR.0000000000000743.

208 Scudiero L, Tak M, Alarcón P, *et al*. Understanding household and food system determinants of chicken and egg consumption in India. *Food Secur*. 2023 Jul 17;15(5):1231-54. doi: 10.1007/s12571-023-01375-3.

209 Zhong VW, Van Horn L, Cornelis MC, *et al*. Associations of dietary cholesterol or egg consumption with incident cardiovascular disease and mortality. *JAMA*. 2019;321(11):1081-95. doi: 10.1001/jama.2019.1572.

210 Kim SR, Kim K, Lee SA, *et al*. Effect of red, processed, and white meat consumption on the risk of gastric cancer: an overall and dose-response meta-analysis. *Nutrients*. 2019;11(4):826. doi: 10.3390/nu11040826.

211 Farvid MS, Stern MC, Norat T, *et al*. Consumption of red and processed meat and breast cancer incidence: a systematic review and meta-analysis of prospective studies. *Int J Cancer*. 2018;143(11):2787-99. doi: 10.1002/ijc.31848.

212 Wolk A. Potential health hazards of eating red meat. *J Intern Med*. 2017;281(2):106-22. doi: 10.1111/joim.12543.

213 Kim K, Hyeon J, Lee SA, Kwon SO, Lee H, *et al*. Role of total, red, processed, and white meat consumption in stroke incidence and

mortality: a systematic review and meta-analysis of prospective cohort studies. *J Am Heart Assoc.* 2017 Aug 30;6(9):e005983. doi:10.1161/JAHA.117.005983. PMID:28855166.

214 Kim Y, Je Y. Meat consumption and risk of metabolic syndrome: results from the Korean population and a meta-analysis of observational studies. *Nutrients.* 2018;10(4):E390. doi: 10.3390/nu10040390.

215 Li C, Bishop TRP, Imamura F, *et al.* Meat consumption and incident type 2 diabetes: an individual-participant federated meta-analysis of 1·97 million adults with 100 000 incident cases from 31 cohorts in 20 countries. *Lancet Diabetes Endocrinol.* 2024 Sep;12(9):619-30. doi: 10.1016/S2213-8587(24)00179-7. PMID: 3917416.

216 Kennedy J, Alexander P, Smith Taillie L, *et al.* Estimated effects of reductions in processed meat consumption and unprocessed red meat consumption on occurrences of type 2 diabetes, cardiovascular disease, colorectal cancer, and mortality in the USA: a microsimulation study. *Lancet Planet Health.* 2024 Jul;8(7):e441-e451. doi: 10.1016/S2542-5196(24)00118-9. PMID: 38969472.

217 Li Y, Li Y, Gu X, Liu Y, Dong D, Kang JH, *et al.* Long-term intake of red meat in relation to dementia risk and cognitive function in US adults. *Neurology.* 2025 Feb 11;104(3):e210286. doi: 10.1212/WNL.0000000000210286.

218 Alexandrov NV, Eelderink C, Singh-Povel CM, *et al.* Dietary protein sources and muscle mass over the life course: the lifelines cohort study. *Nutrients.* 2018;10(10):1471. doi: 10.3390/nu10101471.

219 Jayedi A, Soltani S, Abdolshahi A. Fish consumption and the risk of cardiovascular disease and mortality in patients with type 2 diabetes: a dose-response meta-analysis of prospective cohort studies. *Crit Rev Food Sci Nutr.* 2021;61(10):1640-1650. doi: 10.1080/10408398.2020.1764486.

220 Abdelhamid AS, Brown TJ, Brainard JS, *et al.* Omega-3 fatty acids for the primary and secondary prevention of cardiovascular disease. *Cochrane Database Syst Rev.* 2020;7(17):CD003177.

221 Khan SU, Lone AN, Khan MS, *et al.* Effect of omega-3 fatty acids on cardiovascular outcomes: a systematic review and meta-analysis. *EClinicalMedicine.* 2021;38(5):100997.

222 Sacks FM, Lichtenstein AH, Wu JHY, *et al.* Dietary fats and cardiovascular disease: a presidential advisory from the American Heart Association. *Circulation.* 2017;136(3):e1-e23.

223 Jacobson TA, Glickstein SB, Rowe JD, *et al.* Role of n-3 fatty acids in the treatment of hypertriglyceridemia and cardiovascular disease. *Am J Clin Nutr.* 2008;87(6):1981S-90S. doi: 10.1093/ajcn/87.6.1981S.

224 Bhatt DL, Steg PG, Miller M, *et al.* Cardiovascular risk reduction with icosapent ethyl for hypertriglyceridemia. *N Engl J Med.* 2019;380(1):11–22.

225 Weintraub WS, Goel JR, Hunter P, *et al.* Cost-effectiveness of icosapent ethyl for high-risk patients with hypertriglyceridemia despite statin treatment. *JAMA Netw Open.* 2022;5(2):e2148172.

226 Mozaffarian D, Lemaitre RN, King IB, *et al.* Cardiac benefits of fish consumption may depend on the type of fish meal consumed: the Cardiovascular Health Study. *Circulation.* 2003;107(10):1372–7.

227 Dyall SC, Malau IA, Su KP, *et al.* Omega-3 polyunsaturated fatty acids in depression: insights from recent clinical trials. *Curr Opin Clin Nutr Metab Care.* 2025;28(2):66-74. doi: 10.1097/MCO.0000000000001077.

228 Bisgaard H, Stokholm J, Chawes BL, *et al.* Fish oil-derived fatty acids in pregnancy and wheeze and asthma in offspring. *N Engl J Med.* 2016;375(26):2530–39.

229 Sherzai D, Moness R, Sherzai S, *et al.* A systematic review of omega-3 fatty acid consumption and cognitive outcomes in neurodevelopment. *Am J Lifestyle Med.* 2022;17(5):649-85. doi: 10.1177/15598276221116052.

230 Da Boit M, Sibson R, Sivasubramaniam S, *et al.* Sex differences in the effect of fish-oil supplementation on the adaptive response to resistance exercise training in older people: a randomized controlled trial. *Am J Clin Nutr.* 2017;105(1):151–58.

231 Lin Z, Chen R, Jiang Y, *et al.* Cardiovascular benefits of fish-oil supplementation against fine particulate air pollution in China. *J Am Coll Cardiol.* 2019;73(16):2076–85.

232 Thomsen BJ, Chow EY, Sapijaszko MJ, *et al.* The potential uses of omega-3 fatty acids in dermatology: a review. *J Cutan Med Surg.* 2020;24(5):481-94. doi: 10.1177/1203475420929925.

233 Fatkin D, Cox CD, Martinac B, *et al.* Fishing for links between omega-3 fatty acids and atrial fibrillation. *Circulation.* 2022;145(14):1037-1039. doi: 10.1161/CIRCULATIONAHA.121.058596.

234 Advice about eating fish | FDA [Internet]. Silver Spring (MD): US Food and Drug Administration; [cited 2025 Aug]. Available from: https://www.fda.gov/food/consumers/advice-about-eating-fish.

235 Fraga SRO, Zago L, Curioni CC. Olive oil consumption, risk factors, and diseases: an umbrella review. *Nutr Rev.* 2025 Mar 1;83(3):e1311-e1328. doi: 10.1093/nutrit/nuae091.

236 Fernández del Río L, Gutiérrez-Casado E, Varela-López A, *et al.* Olive oil and the hallmarks of aging. *Molecules.* 2016;21(2):163.

237 Most MM, Tulley R, Morales S, Lefevre M. Rice bran oil, not fiber, lowers cholesterol in humans. *Am J Clin Nutr.* 2005 Jan;81(1):64-8. doi:10.1093/ajcn/81.1.64. PMID:15640461.

238 Hariri Z, Afzalzade F, Sohrab G, Saadati S, Yari Z. The effects of rice bran supplementation for management of blood lipids: a GRADE-assessed systematic review, dose-response meta-analysis, and meta-regression of randomized controlled trials. *Syst Rev.* 2023 Apr 12;12(1):65. doi:10.1186/s13643-023-02228-y.

239 Rezaei S, Akhlaghi M, Sasani MR, *et al.* Olive oil lessened fatty liver severity independent of cardiometabolic correction in patients with non-alcoholic fatty liver disease: a randomized clinical trial. *Nutrition.* 2019 Jan;57:154-61. doi:10.1016/j.nut.2018.02.021. Epub 2018 Mar 23. PMID: 30170304.

240 Nigam P, Bhatt S, Misra A, *et al.* Effect of a 6-month intervention with cooking oils containing a high concentration of monounsaturated fatty acids (olive and canola oils) compared with control oil in male Asian Indians with nonalcoholic fatty liver disease. *Diabetes Technol Ther.* 2014 Apr;16(4):255-61. doi:10.1089/dia.2013.0178. PMID: 24625239.

241 Liu X, Kris-Etherton PM, West SG, Lamarche B, Jenkins DJA, *et al.* Effects of canola and high-oleic-acid canola oils on abdominal fat mass in individuals with central obesity. *Obesity (Silver Spring).* 2016 Nov;24(11):2261-8. doi:10.1002/oby.21584.

242 Mhatre S, Rajaraman P, Chatterjee N, *et al.* Mustard oil consumption, cooking method, diet and gallbladder cancer risk in high- and low-risk regions of India. *Int J Cancer.* 2020 Sep 15;147(6):1621-8. doi:10.1002/ijc.32952. Epub 2020 Mar 30. PMID: 32142159.

243 Dutta U, Bush N, Kalsi D, *et al.* Epidemiology of gallbladder cancer in India. *Chin Clin Oncol.* 2019 Aug;8(4):33. doi:10.21037/cco.2019.08.03. PMID: 31484488.

244 Heid M. Is ghee healthy? Here's what the science says [Internet]. *Time.* 2019 Apr 22 [cited 2025 Aug]. Available from: https://time.com/5571810/is-ghee-healthy/.

245 Odia OJ, Ofori S, Maduka O. Palm oil and the heart: a review. *World J Cardiol.* 2015 Mar 26;7(3):144-149. doi: 10.4330/wjc.v7.i3.144.

246 Ismail SR, Maarof SK, Siedlecki S, *et al.* Systematic review of palm oil consumption and the risk of cardiovascular disease. *PLoS One.* 2018;13(2):e0193533.

247 FSSAI. FSSAI caps trans fatty acids to 2% in all oils & fats by Jan 2022 to prevent thousands of deaths [Internet]. New Delhi: Food Safety and Standards Authority of India; 2021 Jan 8 [cited 2025 Oct].

Available from: https://fssai.gov.in/upload/media/FSSAI_News_Fats_FNB_08_01_2021.pdf.

248 Song P, Jiang Q, Wu X, *et al.* Palmitic acid and palmitoylation in cancer: understanding, insights, and challenges. *The Innovation.* 2025;6(8):100918.

249 Mei J, Qian M, Hou Y, *et al.* Association of saturated fatty acids with cancer risk: a systematic review and meta-analysis. *Lipids Health Dis.* 2024;23(1):32. doi:10.1186/s12944-024-02025-z.

250 Abbasi J. Coconut oil's health halo a mirage, clinical trials suggest. *JAMA.* 2020;323(16):1540-41.

251 Neelakantan N, Seah JYH, van Dam RM, *et al.* The effect of coconut oil consumption on cardiovascular risk factors: a systematic review and meta-analysis of clinical trials. *Circulation.* 2020;141(10):803-14.

252 Jayawardena R, Swarnamali H, Lanerolle P, *et al.* Health effects of coconut oil: summary of evidence from systematic reviews and meta-analysis of interventional studies. *Diabetes Metab Syndr.* 2021;15(2):549-55.

253 Khaw KT, Sharp SJ, Finikarides L, *et al.* Randomised trial of coconut oil, olive oil or butter on blood lipids and other cardiovascular risk factors in healthy men and women. *BMJ Open.* 2018 Mar 6;8(3):e020167. doi:10.1136/bmjopen-2017-020167.

254 Eyres L, Eyres MF, Chisholm A, *et al.* Coconut oil consumption and cardiovascular risk factors in humans. *Nutr Rev.* 2016;74(4):267-80.

255 Faizah O, Merican Z, Hassan MF, *et al.* Effects of consumption of edible oils for a period of 4 months on the ultrastructure of the aorta of spontaneously hypertensive rats. *Asia Pac J Clin Nutr.* 1999;8(2):106-12.

256 Rafique R, Naumana A, Ahmed M. Dietary predictors of early-onset ischaemic heart disease in a sample drawn from a Pakistani population. *Heart Asia.* 2012;4(1):129-34.

257 Ismail J, Jafar TH, Jafary FH, *et al.* Risk factors for non-fatal myocardial infarction in young South Asian adults. *Heart.* 2004;90(3):259-63.

258 Luukkonen PK, Sädevirta S, Zhou Y, *et al.* Saturated fat is more metabolically harmful for the human liver than unsaturated fat or simple sugars. *Diabetes Care.* 2018;41(8):1732-1739.

259 Hosseinabadi SM, Nasrollahzadeh J, Asghari-Jafarabadi M. Effects of diets rich in ghee or olive oil on cardiometabolic risk factors in healthy adults: a two-period, crossover, randomised trial. *Br J Nutr.* 2022;128(9):1720-29.

260 ICMR-NIN Expert Committee. Dietary Guidelines for Indians. Hyderabad: ICMR-National Institute of Nutrition; 2024 [cited 2025 Mar 3]. Available from: https://main.icmr.nic.in/sites/default/files/upload_documents/DGI_07th_May_2024_fin.pdf.

261 Watanabe S, Tsujino S. Applications of medium-chain triglycerides in foods. *Front Nutr.* 2022;9:802805.

262 Sun L, Ye KX, Wong HLK, *et al.* The effects of medium chain triglyceride for Alzheimer's disease related cognitive impairment: a systematic review and meta-analysis. *J Alzheimers Dis.* 2023;94(2):441-56.

263 Ezaki O, Abe S. Medium-chain triglycerides (8:0 and 10:0) increase muscle mass and function in frail older adults: a combined data analysis of clinical trials. *Front Nutr.* 2023;10:1284497.

264 He H, Liu K, Liu M, *et al.* The impact of medium-chain triglycerides on weight loss and metabolic health in individuals with overweight or obesity: a systematic review and meta-analysis. *Clin Nutr.* 2024;43(8):1755-68.

265 Garg A, Bonanome A, Grundy SM, *et al.* Comparison of a high-carbohydrate diet with a high-monounsaturated-fat diet in patients with non-insulin-dependent diabetes mellitus. *N Engl J Med.* 1988 Sep 29;319(13):829-34. doi:10.1056/NEJM198809293191304.

266 Mancini A, Imperlini E, Nigro E, *et al.* Biological and nutritional properties of palm oil and palmitic acid: effects on health. *Molecules.* 2015;20(9):17339–61. doi:10.3390/molecules200917339.

267 Bukhari DA, Faheem M, Arshad S, *et al.* Effect of high dietary consumption of locally available ghee on renal function in mice. *Pak J Zool.* 2020;52(3):901-909. doi:10.17582/journal.pjz/20190623160652.

268 Hosseini M, Adimi Naghan P, Moghadas Jafari A, *et al.* Nutrition and lung cancer: a case control study in Iran. *BMC Cancer.* 2014 Nov 21;14:860. doi:10.1186/1471-2407-14-860. PMID:25416035.

269 Gulati S, Misra A. Sugar intake, obesity, and diabetes in India. *Nutrients.* 2014;6(12):5955-74. doi:10.3390/nu6125955.

270 Touvier M, da Costa Louzada ML, Mozaffarian D, *et al.* Ultra-processed foods and cardiometabolic health: public health policies to reduce consumption cannot wait. *BMJ.* 2023 Oct 10;383:e075294. doi: 10.1136/bmj-2023-075294.

271 Malik VS, Hu FB. Sugar-sweetened beverages and cardiometabolic health: an update of the evidence. *Nutrients.* 2019;11(8):1840. doi:10.3390/nu11081840.

272 Lara-Castor L, O'Hearn M, Cudhea F, *et al.* Burdens of type 2 diabetes and cardiovascular disease attributable to sugar-sweetened beverages in 184 countries. *Nat Med.* 2025;31:552-64. doi:10.1038/s41591-024-xxxxx-x.

273 Jones T, Dunn EL, Macdonald JH, *et al.* The effects of beetroot juice on blood pressure, microvascular function and large-vessel endothelial function: a randomized, double-blind, placebo-controlled pilot study

in healthy older adults. *Nutrients*. 2019;11(8):1792. doi:10.3390/nu11081792.

274 Maki KC, Kaspar KL, Khoo C, *et al.* Consumption of a cranberry juice beverage lowered the number of clinical urinary tract infection episodes in women with a recent history of urinary tract infection. *Am J Clin Nutr.* 2016;103(6):1434-42. doi:10.3945/ajcn.116.130542.

275 Kerimi A, Nyambe-Silavwe H, Gauer JS, *et al.* Pomegranate juice, but not an extract, confers a lower glycemic response on a high-glycemic index food: randomized, crossover, controlled trials in healthy subjects. *Am J Clin Nutr.* 2017;106(6):1384-93. doi:10.3945/ajcn.117.161968.

276 Ghavipour M, Saedisomeolia A, Djalali M, *et al.* Tomato juice consumption improves blood antioxidative biomarkers in overweight and obese females. *Clin Nutr.* 2015;34(5):805-9. doi:10.1016/j.clnu.2014.10.012.

277 World Health Organization. WHO advises not to use non-sugar sweeteners for weight control in newly released guideline [Internet]. Geneva:WHO; 2023 [cited 2025 Mar 3]. Available from: https://www.who.int/news/item/15-05-2023-who-advises-not-to-use-non-sugar-sweeteners-for-weight-control-in-newly-released-guideline.

278 Singh A, Singh A, Singh R, *et al.* Non-sugar sweeteners and health outcomes in adults without diabetes: deciphering the WHO recommendations in the Indian context. *Diabetes Metab Syndr.* 2023;17(8):102829. doi:10.1016/j.dsx.2023.102829.

279 Zhang R, Noronha JC, Khan TA, *et al.* The effect of non-nutritive sweetened beverages on postprandial glycemic and endocrine responses: a systematic review and network meta-analysis. *Nutrients.* 2023 Feb 20;15(4):1050. doi: 10.3390/nu15041050.

280 Toews I, Lohner S, Küllenberg de Gaudry D, *et al.* Association between intake of non-sugar sweeteners and health outcomes: systematic review and meta-analyses of randomised and non-randomised controlled trials and observational studies. *BMJ.* 2019 Jan 2;364:k4718. doi: 10.1136/bmj.k4718.

281 Debras C, Chazelas E, Srour B, *et al.* Artificial sweeteners and cancer risk: results from the NutriNet-Santé population-based cohort study. *PLoS Med.* 2022 Mar 24;19(3):e1003950. doi: 10.1371/journal.pmed.1003950.

282 Witkowski M, Nemet I, Alamri H, *et al.* The artificial sweetener erythritol and cardiovascular event risk. *Nat Med.* 2023 Mar;29(3):710-18. doi: 10.1038/s41591-023-02223-9.

283 Debras C, Chazelas E, Sellem L, *et al.* Artificial sweeteners and risk of cardiovascular diseases: results from the prospective NutriNet-Santé cohort. *BMJ.* 2022 Sep 7;378:e071204. doi: 10.1136/bmj-2022-071204.

284 Debras C, Deschasaux-Tanguy M, Chazelas E, *et al.* Artificial sweeteners and risk of type 2 diabetes in the prospective NutriNet-Santé cohort. *Diabetes Care.* 2023;46(9):1681–90. doi:10.2337/dc23-0206.

285 Gregory A. Artificial sweeteners linked to increased risk of heart disease, study finds [Internet]. London: *Guardian*; 2022 Sep 7 [cited 2025 Oct 10]. Available from: https://www.theguardian.com/society/2022/sep/07/artificial-sweeteners-linked-to-increased-risk-of-heart-disease-study-finds.

286 Bahrami M, Ataie-Jafari A, Hosseini S, *et al.* Effects of natural honey consumption in diabetic patients: an 8-week randomized clinical trial. *Int J Food Sci Nutr.* 2009;60(7):618-26. doi: 10.3109/09637480801990389.

287 Ramli NZ, Chin KY, Zarkasi KA, *et al.* A review on the protective effects of honey against metabolic syndrome. *Nutrients.* 2018 Aug 2;10(8):1009. doi: 10.3390/nu10081009.

288 Münstedt K, Sheybani B, Hauenschild A, *et al.* Effects of basswood honey, honey-comparable glucose-fructose solution, and oral glucose tolerance test solution on serum insulin, glucose, and C-peptide concentrations in healthy subjects. *J Med Food.* 2008 Sep;11(3):424-8. doi: 10.1089/jmf.2007.0608.

289 Hung CT. Effects of high-fructose (90%) corn syrup on plasma glucose, insulin, and c-peptide in non-insulin-dependent diabetes mellitus and normal subjects. *Taiwan Yi Xue Hui Za Zhi.* 1989;88(9):883-85.

290 Chung M, Ma J, Patel K, *et al.* Fructose, high-fructose corn syrup, sucrose, and non-alcoholic fatty liver disease or indexes of liver health: a systematic review and meta-analysis. *Am J Clin Nutr.* 2014;100(3):833-49. doi: 10.3945/ajcn.114.086314.

291 DeChristopher LR, Tucker KL. Disproportionately higher cardiovascular disease risk and incidence with high fructose corn syrup sweetened beverage intake among black young adults-the CARDIA study. *Nutr J.* 2024 Jul 29;23(1):84. doi: 10.1186/s12937-024-00978-6.

292 Li J, Chen XL, Ou-Yang XL, *et al.* Association of tea consumption with all-cause/cardiovascular disease mortality in the chronic kidney disease population: an assessment of participation in the national cohort. *Ren Fail.* 2025 Dec;47(1):2449578. doi: 10.1080/0886022X.2025.2449578. Epub 2025 Jan 13.

293 Larsson SC. Coffee, tea, and cocoa and risk of stroke. *Stroke.* 2014;45(1):309-14. doi: 10.1161/STROKEAHA.113.003131.

294 Yi M, Wu X, Zhuang W, *et al.* Tea consumption and health outcomes: umbrella review of meta-analyses of observational studies in humans. *Mol Nutr Food Res.* 2019;63(16):e1900389. doi: 10.1002/mnfr.201900389.

295 Samavat H, Newman AR, Wang R, *et al.* Effects of green tea catechin extract on serum lipids in postmenopausal women: a randomized, placebo-controlled clinical trial. *Am J Clin Nutr.* 2016;104(6):1671-82. doi: 10.3945/ajcn.116.144972.

296 Zamani M, Kelishadi MR, Ashtary-Larky D, *et al.* The effects of green tea supplementation on cardiovascular risk factors: a systematic review and meta-analysis. *Front Nutr.* 2023 Jan 10;9:1084455. doi: 10.3389/fnut.2022.1084455. eCollection 2022.

297 Jurgens TM, Whelan AM, Killian L, *et al.* Green tea for weight loss and weight maintenance in overweight or obese adults. *Cochrane Database Syst Rev.* 2012;12(12):CD008650. doi: 10.1002/14651858.CD008650.pub2.

298 Kakutani S, Watanabe H, Murayama N, *et al.* Green tea intake and risks for dementia, Alzheimer's disease, mild cognitive impairment, and cognitive impairment: a systematic review. *Nutrients.* 2019;11(5):1165. doi: 10.3390/nu11051165.

299 Yoneshiro T, Matsushita M, Hibi M, *et al.* Tea catechin and caffeine activate brown adipose tissue and increase cold-induced thermogenic capacity in humans. *Am J Clin Nutr.* 2017;105(4):873-81. doi: 10.3945/ajcn.116.144972.

300 Luk HY, Appell C, Chyu MC, *et al.* Impacts of green tea on joint and skeletal muscle health: prospects of translational nutrition. *Antioxidants (Basel).* 2020 Oct 28;9(11):1050. doi: 10.3390/antiox9111050.

301 Ide K, Kawasaki Y, Akutagawa M, *et al.* Effects of green tea gargling on the prevention of influenza infection: an analysis using Bayesian approaches. *J Altern Complement Med.* 2017 Feb;23(2):116-20. doi: 10.1089/acm.2016.0094.

302 Ota N, Soga S, Shimotoyodome A, *et al.* Daily consumption of tea catechins improves aerobic capacity in healthy male adults: a randomized double-blind, placebo-controlled, crossover trial. *Biosci Biotechnol Biochem.* 2016;80(12):2412-17. doi: 10.1089/acm.2016.0094.

303 Butacnum A, Chongsuwat R, Bumrungpert A. Black tea consumption improves postprandial glycemic control in normal and pre-diabetic subjects: a randomized, double-blind, placebo-controlled crossover study. *Asia Pac J Clin Nutr.* 2017 Jan;26(1):59-64. doi: 10.6133/apjcn.112015.08.

304 Latif R. Chocolate/cocoa and human health: a review. *Neth J Med.* 2013;71(2):63-68.

305 Leyva-Soto X, Chavez-Santoscoy RA, Lara-Jacobo LR, *et al.* Daily consumption of chocolate rich in flavonoids decreases cellular genotoxicity and improves biochemical parameters of lipid and

glucose metabolism. *Molecules*. 2018;23(9):E2220. doi:10.3390/molecules23092220.

306 West SG, McIntyre MD, Piotrowski MJ, *et al.* Effects of dark chocolate and cocoa consumption on endothelial function and arterial stiffness in overweight adults. *Br J Nutr.* 2014;111(4):653-61. doi:10.1017/S0007114513002912.

307 Pereira T, Bergqvist J, Vieira C, *et al.* Randomized study of the effects of cocoa-rich chocolate on the ventricle-arterial coupling and vascular function of young, healthy adults. *Nutrition*. 2019;63-64:175-83. doi:10.1016/j.nut.2019.02.017.

308 Hollands WJ, Tapp H, Defernez M, *et al.* Lack of acute or chronic effects of epicatechin-rich and procyanidin-rich apple extracts on blood pressure and cardiometabolic biomarkers in adults with moderately elevated blood pressure: a randomized, placebo-controlled crossover trial. *Am J Clin Nutr.* 2018;108(5):1006-1014. doi:10.1093/ajcn/nqy139.

309 Zhao B, Gan L, Yu K, *et al.* Relationship between chocolate consumption and overall and cause-specific mortality, systematic review and updated meta-analysis. *Eur J Epidemiol.* 2022;37(4):321-33. doi:10.1007/s10654-022-00858-5.

310 Liu B, Zong G, Zhu L, *et al.* Chocolate intake and risk of type 2 diabetes: prospective cohort studies. *BMJ*. 2024;387:e078386. doi:10.1136/bmj-2023-078386.

311 Malhi H, Loomba R. Editorial: dark chocolate may improve NAFLD and metabolic syndrome by reducing oxidative stress. *Aliment Pharmacol Ther.* 2016;44(5):533-4. doi:10.1111/apt.13716.

312 Marsh CE, Green DJ, Naylor LH, *et al.* Consumption of dark chocolate attenuates subsequent food intake compared with milk and white chocolate in postmenopausal women. *Appetite.* 2017;116:544-51.

313 Behzadi M, Vesal Bideshki M, Ahmadi-Khorram M, *et al.* Effect of dark chocolate/cocoa consumption on oxidative stress and inflammation in adults: a GRADE-assessed systematic review and dose-response meta-analysis of controlled trials. *Complement Ther Med.* 2024;84:103061. doi:10.1016/j.ctim.2024.103061.:10.1016/j.appet.2017.05.050.

314 Mostofsky E, Berg Johansen M, Tjønneland A, *et al.* Chocolate intake and risk of clinically apparent atrial fibrillation: the Danish diet, cancer, and health study. *Heart.* 2017;103(15):1163-7. doi:10.1136/heartjnl-2016-310357.

315 Liu H, Ye M, Guo H, *et al.* An updated review of randomized clinical trials testing the improvement of cognitive function of ginkgo biloba extract in healthy people and Alzheimer's patients. *Front Pharmacol.* 2020;10:1688. doi: 10.3389/fphar.2019.01688.

316 Lin J, Sun X, Yang L, *et al.* Effects and safety of ginkgo biloba on depression: a systematic review and meta-analysis. *Front Pharmacol.* 2024 Mar 18;15:1364030. doi: 10.3389/fphar.2024.1364030.

317 Sereda M, Xia J, Scutt P, *et al.* Ginkgo biloba for tinnitus. *Cochrane Database Syst Rev.* 2022 Nov 16;2022(11):CD013514. doi: 10.1002/14651858.CD013514.pub2.

318 Abebe W. Review of herbal medications with the potential to cause bleeding: dental implications, and risk prediction and prevention avenues. *EPMA J.* 2019 Jan 8;10(1):51-64. doi: 10.1007/s13167-018-0158-2.

319 Mei N, Guo X, Ren Z, *et al.* Review of ginkgo biloba-induced toxicity, from experimental studies to human case reports. *J Environ Sci Health C Environ Carcinog Ecotoxicol Rev.* 2017;35(1):1-28. doi: 10.1080/10590501.2016.1278298.

320 Yagnik D, Serafin V, Shah AJ. Antimicrobial activity of apple cider vinegar against *Escherichia coli, Staphylococcus aureus* and *Candida albicans*; downregulating cytokine and microbial protein expression. *Sci Rep.* 2018;8(1):1732. doi: 10.1038/s41598-017-18618-x.

321 Petsiou EI, Mitrou PI, Raptis SA, *et al.* Effect and mechanisms of action of vinegar on glucose metabolism, lipid profile, and body weight. *Nutr Rev.* 2014;72(10):651-61. doi: 10.1111/nure.12125.

322 van Dijk JW, Tummers K, Hamer HM, *et al.* Vinegar co-ingestion does not improve oral glucose tolerance in patients with type 2 diabetes. *J Diabetes Complications.* 2012;26(5):460-61. doi: 10.1016/j.jdiacomp.2012.05.009.

323 Liatis S, Grammatikou S, Poulia KA, *et al.* Vinegar reduces postprandial hyperglycaemia in patients with type ii diabetes when added to a high, but not to a low, glycaemic index meal. *Eur J Clin Nutr.* 2010;64(7):727-32. doi: 10.1038/ejcn.2010.89.

324 Hadi A, Pourmasoumi M, Najafgholizadeh A, *et al.* The effect of apple cider vinegar on lipid profiles and glycemia parameters: a systematic review and meta-analysis of randomised clinical trials. *BMC Complement Med Ther.* 2021;21:179. doi: 10.1186/s12906-021-03351-w.

325 Hill LL, Woodruff LH, Foote JC, *et al.* Esophageal injury by apple cider vinegar tablets and subsequent evaluation of products. *J Am Diet Assoc.* 2005;105(7):1141-44.

326 Lhotta K, Höfle G, Gasser R, *et al.* Hypokalemia, hyperreninemia and osteoporosis in a patient ingesting large amounts of cider vinegar. *Nephron.* 1998 Oct;80(2):242-3. doi: 10.1159/000045180.

327 Hlebowicz J, Darwiche G, Björgell O, *et al.* Effect of apple cider vinegar on delayed gastric emptying in patients with type 1 diabetes mellitus: a pilot study. *BMC Gastroenterol.* 2007 Dec 20;7:46. doi: 10.1186/1471-230X-7-46.

328 Arring NM, Millstine D, Marks LA, *et al.* Ginseng as a treatment for fatigue: a systematic review. *J Altern Complement Med.* 2018;24(7):624-33. doi:10.1089/acm.2017.0361.

329 Shergis JL, Thien F, Worsnop CJ, *et al.* 12-month randomised controlled trial of ginseng extract for moderate COPD. *Thorax.* 2019;74(6):539-45. doi:10.1136/thoraxjnl-2018-212665.

330 Seida JK, Durec T, Kuhle S. North American (*Panax quinquefolius*) and Asian Ginseng (*Panax ginseng*) preparations for prevention of the common cold in healthy adults: a systematic review. *Evid Based Complement Alternat Med.* 2011;2011:282151. doi:10.1093/ecam/nep068.

331 Cho YH, Ahn SC, Lee SY, *et al.* Effect of Korean red ginseng on insulin sensitivity in non-diabetic healthy overweight and obese adults. *Asia Pac J Clin Nutr.* 2013;22(3):365-71. doi:10.6133/apjcn.2013.22.3.04.

332 Kim SY, Seo SK, Choi YM, *et al.* Effects of red ginseng supplementation on menopausal symptoms and cardiovascular risk factors in postmenopausal women: a double-blind randomized controlled trial. *Menopause.* 2012;19(4):461-6. doi:10.1097/gme.0b013e3182325e4b.

333 Cardinal BJ, Engels HJ, Zhu W. Ginseng does not enhance psychological well-being in healthy, young adults: results of a double-blind, placebo-controlled, randomized clinical trial. *J Am Diet Assoc.* 2001;101(6):655-60.

334 Ghorbani Z, Mirghafourvand M, Mohammad-Alizadeh Charandabi S, *et al.* The effect of ginseng on sexual dysfunction in menopausal women: a double-blind, randomized, controlled trial. *Complement Ther Med.* 2019;45:57-64. doi:10.1016/j.ctim.2019.05.015.

335 Liu L. Side effects of ginseng supplements [Internet]. Washington (DC): National Capital Poison Center; [cited 2025 Mar]. Available from: https://www.poison.org/articles/side-effects-of-ginseng-supplements-191.

Chapter 6 Supplements and Vitamins

1 Middha P, Weinstein SJ, Männistö S, *et al.* β-Carotene supplementation and lung cancer incidence in the Alpha-Tocopherol, Beta-Carotene Cancer Prevention Study: the role of tar and nicotine. *Nicotine Tob Res.* 2018;21(8):1045-1050. doi: 10.1093/ntr/nty115.

2 Ronis MJJ, Pedersen KB, Watt J. Adverse effects of nutraceuticals and dietary supplements. *Annu Rev Pharmacol Toxicol.* 2018;58:583-601. doi: 10.1146/annurev-pharmtox-010617-052844. Epub 2017 Oct 6. PMID: 28992429.

3 Bhatt SP, Misra A, Pandey RM, *et al.* Vitamin D supplementation in overweight/obese Asian Indian women with prediabetes reduces

glycemic measures and truncal subcutaneous fat: a 78 weeks randomized placebo-controlled trial (PREVENT-WIN trial). *Sci Rep*. 2020;10(1):220. doi: 10.1038/s41598-019-56904-y.

4 Gagnon C, Daly RM, Carpentier A, *et al.* Effects of combined calcium and vitamin D supplementation on insulin secretion, insulin sensitivity and β-cell function in multi-ethnic vitamin D-deficient adults at risk for type 2 diabetes: a pilot randomized, placebo-controlled trial. *PLoS One*. 2014;9(10):e109607. doi: 10.1371/journal.pone.0109607.

5 ICMR-NIN Expert Committee. Dietary Guidelines for Indians. Hyderabad: ICMR-National Institute of Nutrition; 2024 [cited 2025 Mar 3]. Available from: https://main.icmr.nic.in/sites/default/files/upload_documents/DGI_07th_May_2024_fin.pdf.

6 Anoop Misra. *Diabetes with Delight*. New Delhi: Bloomsbury India; 2018.

About the Author

Dr Anoop Misra is chairman of the Fortis C-DOC Centre of Excellence for Diabetes, Metabolic Diseases and Endocrinology in New Delhi, and director of both the National Diabetes, Obesity and Cholesterol Foundation and the Diabetes Foundation (India). He trained at the All India Institute of Medical Sciences (AIIMS), New Delhi, and subsequently worked at leading institutions in London and at the UT Southwestern Medical Center in Dallas, US.

Over the past four decades, Dr Misra has played a defining role in advancing diabetes care in India—as a clinician, researcher, teacher and national advisor. He has served on major committees addressing diabetes, obesity, fatty liver disease and nutrition, and has advised key national bodies, including the Ministry of Health, the National Institute of Nutrition, the Indian Council of Medical Research, the Department of Health Research, the Ministry of Health and Family Welfare and the Niti Aayog, Government of India.

A prolific scientist, Dr Misra has published more than 400 research papers and several book chapters. His work is widely cited and has significantly shaped the global understanding of obesity, diabetes and nutrition in Indian populations. Analyses from Stanford University (2022–2024) ranked him among the top 2 per cent of scientists worldwide in diabetes research and in 2023, he was identified as the top-ranked researcher in diabetes and endocrinology in India.

Dr Misra is the editor-in-chief of *Diabetes & Metabolic Syndrome: Clinical Research & Reviews*. He serves on the editorial advisory board of the *British Medical Journal*, is part of its regional advisory board for South Asia and its academic commission, and has also been a member of the Lancet Obesity Commission (2024–2025). In 2024, he was elected to Sigma Xi, the prestigious US research honor society.

His clinical and research contributions have been widely recognised through major awards, including the Dr B.C. Roy

Award, India's highest medical honour, and the Padma Shri, one of India's highest civilian honours. His current research interests span diabetes and prediabetes, diet, metabolism, clinical nutrition, liver and pancreatic fat, muscle health, and the relationship between vitamin D, metabolism and longevity.

Deeply committed to equitable healthcare, Dr Misra leads the outreach initiative Diabetes Care at Doorsteps, which has delivered services to nearly 2,00,000 underprivileged individuals in Delhi. He strongly advocates recognising obesity as a chronic disease and continues to pursue practical, innovative solutions for prevention and care.

He is also the author of the bestselling books *Diabetes with Delight* and *Diabetes Ke Saath Khushhaal Jeevan*, published by Bloomsbury.